Praise for Mara Schiavocampo's
THINspired

"The best weight-loss book you'll ever read and need to keep the pounds off."

—*Hello Beautiful*

"Mara's bright smile and sharp reporting have always stood out, but as I've watched her life and career blossom, I've been amazed watching her physically transform as well. She has always been a beautiful person inside and out—but after reading this book, she will truly inspire you to be the best version of yourself. Go Mara go!"

—Amy Robach, news anchor, *Good Morning America*

"I thought I had read just about everything as it comes to living a healthy lifestyle. Then I read Mara's story and was immediately inspired. Who knew she was so funny? I laughed. I cried. I lost 10 pounds."

—Don Lemon, cohost of *CNN Tonight*

"I've lost 15 pounds in 2 months using Mara's common sense advice. No jokes. No gimmicks. *THINspired* is easy to read, accessible, and REAL. This is the book to read if you are interested in losing weight and keeping it off. Her story is inspiring. A MUST-READ."

—Amanda Johnson

"Loved, loved . . . LOVED this book. I feel so inspired by Mara's words and I feel like I know her personally! She's real . . .she's funny, and she's right!"

—M. Garcia

"This is such an amazing book. Everything she says is so real. If you follow her advice, you will lose weight. I lost 18 pounds already."

—Angela F.

"It's like having a sorority sister as your personal lifestyle coach as you embrace a new way of eating and living. This is one I'll be rereading frequently."

—EJG

"*THINspired* is a great read as part of an overall plan to get healthy. It's full of tips and recipes that help with your game plan. It was sold out when I went to my local bookstore to get a copy. Seriously, get yours before they run out."

—R. Clark

"This book has renewed my sense of dedication to MYSELF and has motivated me to get back up again! 'Mara's formula' is so simple, so logical, that it had me sitting there staring at it thinking 'Wow. THAT is IT.'"

—L. Pav

"I would really like to say a big thank-you to Mara, you are inspiring me without making me feel bad about myself. This book gives you the info you need to make the changes you need to with some good scientific findings and the findings of a person who is just like all of us and has struggles but yet succeeded."

—Bakery Chick

THINspired

How I Lost 90 Pounds

My Plan for
Lasting Weight Loss and
Self-Acceptance

MARA SCHIAVOCAMPO

GALLERY BOOKS | KAREN HUNTER PUBLISHING
New York London Toronto Sydney New Delhi

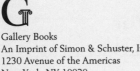

Gallery Books
An Imprint of Simon & Schuster, Inc.
1230 Avenue of the Americas
New York, NY 10020

Karen Hunter Publishing,
A Division of Suitt-Hunter Enterprises, LLC
P.O. Box 632
South Orange, NJ 07079

First Karen Hunter Publishing/Gallery Books trade paperback edition January 2016

GALLERY and colophon are registered trademarks of Simon & Schuster, Inc.

For information about special discounts for bulk purchases,
please contact Simon & Schuster Special Sales at
1-866-506-1949 or business@simonandschuster.com.

The Simon & Schuster Speakers Bureau can bring authors to your live event. For
more information or to book an event contact the Simon & Schuster Speakers
Bureau at 1-866-248-3049 or visit our website at www.simonspeakers.com.

Interior design by Julie Schroeder

Manufactured in the United States of America

10 9 8 7 6 5 4 3 2 1

Library of Congress Cataloging-in-Publication Data for the hardcover edition
is available.

ISBN 978-1-4767-8405-2
ISBN 978-1-4767-8406-9 (pbk)
ISBN 978-1-4767-8408-3 (ebook)

To my precious Nina Bella.
The day your life began, so too did mine.

Contents

— CONTENTS —

THINspired

Introduction

Imagine waking up one morning and being thin. Wait, let's back up a minute. First, imagine having a lifelong history of weight problems, dating back to childhood, spending decades agonizing over what to eat and how much you weigh, struggling like hell to lose even an ounce, and being ninety pounds overweight. *Now* imagine waking up one morning and being thin. Sound impossible? Well, it happened to me.

Okay, so it wasn't *exactly* like that, but I wanted to get your attention. What actually happened is that I started making small, incremental changes in my life, things that in some ways were almost imperceptible. Once I got used to one, I'd make another. All the while, I went on about my life. I wasn't agonizing. I didn't spend every meal adding up a different set of numbers, from calories, to carbs, to points. I just lived.

Some of the changes involved food. Some involved exercise. Some had nothing to do with either one of those things, but contributed to my overall happiness. I spent a lot of time focusing on *my* happiness. How great is that?

I'm not a completely clueless dope, so of course I noticed changes. My clothes started fitting better. I'd step on the scale and go "ooh," instead of "ugh." When I would give myself a break and indulge in some of my old favorite snacks, they'd kind of make me nauseous, which is never the feeling you want from your comfort food. So, yes, I knew something was afoot. But I had no clue to what degree.

One day, I saw a photo of myself and thought, *Whoa. I'm thin.* I was floored. I simply could not believe that girl was me. She wasn't "thick" or "curvy," and definitely not plus-sized. She was *thin.* And her arms had like, some definition to them. *When the hell did that happen?* I thought to myself.

That night I looked through my closet and realized that almost everything was a size medium or 8, and much of it was too big. In the past, the smallest thing in my closet was a size 12 (not counting that one pair of aspirational skinny jeans from college tucked in the back). I was genuinely perplexed. *If everything in my closet is a size 8, does that make me a size 8?* I thought, scratching my head like a caveman. *Wait . . . one . . . minute. If everything in my closet is too big at a size 8, does that make me a size 6?!* I'm slow, but eventually I'll get there.

Math has never been my strong suit, but these observations forced me to surrender. I started counting how many pounds I'd lost. See, when I was stepping on the scale all those months, it mostly just triggered a trip down memory lane.

"Oh, there's my pre-baby weight."

"I haven't seen this weight since college."

"Now that's a new number!" and so forth.

My goals were always in three- to five-pound increments, so I wasn't keeping track of a grand total. Now, faced with all of this mounting evidence of a huge weight loss, I had to add it up. I knew the general ballpark, more or less, but the final tally still shocked me: ninety pounds. I'd lost ninety pounds. At first I thought I'd done the math wrong, which for me is more than likely. But after several checks and rechecks, the number always came up the same. It felt unreal. So while it's true that my journey didn't happen overnight, in a lot of ways the realization did.

That's my story. Now let's get to you, because something tells me that if you're reading this book, you want to be accidentally thin, too. When I first lost the weight, several times a week I'd get asked the same question: "What are you doing?!" I'd get emails from viewers and old friends alike. Coworkers would stop me in the halls. At first, I really had to think hard about how to answer that question, because, like I mentioned, it all just kind of *happened*. But when I stopped to focus on what I'd done and how I'd done it, I realized that there was in fact a method to the madness, a formula if you will, that led me to the life that had eluded me for so long.

One bit of sober wisdom before we embark on this journey: While you may become aware of your progress overnight, like I did, this is most certainly not a quick fix. If that's what you're looking for, you may want to go and drink cabbage soup for a week. This is about a slow, gradual *lifestyle* change. It's not a sprint. It's a marathon. The good news is, if you're truly changing your lifestyle, you only have to do it once. It's been said that the journey of a thousand miles begins with a single step. It's time to put that first foot forward.

Chapter I

MEMORY LANE
From the Beginning

All right, guys, get your violins out. My history with weight issues isn't exactly cheery. I'll start by saying this, though: I never feel sad or angry when I think of any of what I'm about to share. I fully subscribe to the belief that everything I'm not makes me everything I am. It's all part of what makes me, me.

Like so many kids who grew up in the 1980s, I spent Saturday mornings binge-watching cartoons. At the risk of sounding like an old grump, we didn't have it as easy as kids today. There were no cartoons on demand through YouTube, or twenty-four-hour cable channels like the Cartoon Network. None of that. You pretty much had one window for all of your prime kid shows, and it was Saturday morning. My siblings and I would wake up well before my parents, rush to the family room, and camp out under the TV for hours. It was about as good as it gets.

Unfortunately for me, those mornings were always bittersweet. Most weeks, at some point during our cartoon-a-thon, I would get called away. As soon as I heard my name being shouted from a neighboring room, my stomach would clench into knots. I wished I could run away and hide. I thought maybe if I ignored the call, it would go away. But that never worked. It was time for my weekly weigh-in.

As part of a family member's loving but misguided attempt to help me shed baby fat, each week I was summoned to stand on the scale. Let's call this family member Aunt Shirley. Aunt Shirley firmly believed that a woman—or young girl, for that matter—would never be happy if she was overweight, destined to be completely ostracized from society, like a modern-day leper.

"You'll never have a boyfriend if you're fat," she'd say. "No one will want to be friends with you. You'll get picked on at school."

While I was indeed a little bit chubby, I was by no means fat. At nine years old, I was your pretty typical "round" kid. But Aunt Shirley saw my roundness as the early stages of obesity and was determined to stop it.

The weigh-ins were designed not just to monitor my weight, but also to motivate me to drop pounds. The problem is, as a kid, I really had no idea how one lost weight. Sure, I knew it had to do with food and exercise, but just in broad terms. As far as I was concerned, whether I gained or lost weight that week was due to the luck of the draw. It seemed like pure chance. So I'd take a deep breath, step on the scale, and hope for the best.

Some weeks I lost weight, and some weeks I gained. When the number dropped, I felt like a huge *psychological* weight had been lifted as well. Aunt Shirley would smile in vindication, as proud of herself as she was of me, thinking her approach was finally working. I felt a sense of pride myself, as though I'd actually accomplished something in being lucky that week. Adding to the glory of the moment was the relief that I knew I was as far as possible from my next weigh-in the following weekend. And to top it all off, I would get a reward. Are you ready for this? Perversely, my prize was often food. Aunt Shirley would proclaim that I would be allowed to have ice cream for dessert that night, or some such treat. How's that for confusing? To put it mildly, Aunt Shirley was far from perfect.

Then there were the weeks when I'd gain. To this day, those were among the most humiliating moments of my life. I felt an overwhelming sense of shame; guilty of a terrible sin, publicly revealed. In those minutes I felt so very small, exposed, vulnerable, and utterly worthless. All I wanted was to disappear. Aunt Shirley would look so disappointed. She would scowl and shake her head as if to say, "What's wrong with this child?" That's often when she would regale me with her predictions of a fat and lonely future. Then I would learn of the consequences. Weight loss came with a reward. Gaining led to a penalty. Most often I would have my allowance taken away for the week. But the real punishment had already taken place, in the way those moments made me feel.

Aunt Shirley's weight loss plan didn't end with the scale. It was a near-constant system of pressure. At dinner, she would scold me for eating too much. She'd call me "House" (as in, "big as a house") *while* I was eating, as though it was my name. "Another serving, House?"

If she found the remnants of an unhealthy snack

in the cupboard or fridge, she'd bring it directly to me for a confrontation. "Is this yours?" she'd ask. "Do you know how many calories this has? Don't you know eating this stuff will make you fat? What are you thinking?" She was utterly obsessed with controlling my food. There was never a reprieve, not even on Thanksgiving. "Pie?! You're having pie?"

In hindsight, as an adult, I can see that Aunt Shirley, being obese herself, was dealing with issues that went far beyond me. She was phenomenally undisciplined about her own food, often eating like a medieval king. It was far easier to place an iron grip on my habits than lead by example and change her own. But as a kid, I thought it was all my fault. I wore shame like a second skin. Let's just say I developed a complicated relationship with food and my weight.

The thing is, I was a headstrong kid, and after a few years of this torment, I went from shame alone to resistance as well, rebelling against Aunt Shirley's oppression by secretly bingeing. This was my guerrilla warfare, undermining the obligatory diets by eating junk as often as possible, but always in private. I would tiptoe into enemy territory (the kitchen), sneak food back to the bunker (my bedroom), and launch my secret assault, scarfing down whatever

I'd been able to steal, from doughnuts to chips to an entire can of cake frosting all by itself, scooping it up with my bare fingers. It wasn't about the food. It was about control. Those binges became such a comfort; brief vacations from what felt like daily monitoring of every morsel I put into my mouth, most often followed by a lecture. I learned that there was only one way to really relax: Eat. A lot.

Eating without being watched, monitored, or scolded was absolutely blissful. There was the pleasure of the food, the freedom from Aunt Shirley's control, and the symbolic middle finger I was extending her way. It was intoxicating, and it became my drug while I was still just a child.

The weigh-ins finally stopped when I hit middle school, after I learned how a scale worked in science class. The teacher explained that a key component of the scale was the metal spring inside. That afternoon I went home, unscrewed the back of the scale, and lo and behold, a spring! I took it out and put the scale back together. It worked like a charm; when I stepped on the scale the needle didn't move the slightest bit. I might as well have been made of air. Mission accomplished! That Saturday during my weigh-in, Aunt Shirley looked perplexed, but she let me off the hook. Much to my great relief, she never got around to buying another scale.

By the time I graduated from high school, I was a size 14. Not large by any stretch; in fact, that's the size of the average American woman today. But at five feet three, I was definitely plus-sized, and by no means thin. Aunt Shirley's harassment continued until the moment I left for college, as did my binge-ing. It's no wonder I went clear across the country for school.

When I arrived at the University of California from Maryland, I quickly learned there's no better motivation to get in shape than living someplace where the sun shines every day! I wanted to wear shorts and tank tops year-round, just like the other girls. Aunt Shirley wasn't around, so there was really no reason to binge. I had no one to rebel against. Plus, I was having a ball. Who needs to self-medicate when you're living with all of your best girlfriends on one of the most beautiful college campuses in the country, going to class fifteen hours a week and partying all the time? I started eating less and less. I exercised. I lost twenty-five pounds and slipped into single-digit sizes. I was surprised by how easy it was. *I've beat this thing*, I thought, dusting my hands off, inner demons vanquished. Alas, there's this funny thing about those demons: While we're proclaiming victory, they're out back doing push-ups.

After graduation I landed what seemed like a dream job in New York as a reporter and anchor for a national college television network. My first on-air gig, the position came with a decent salary and lots of perks, including a seasonal allowance for clothes and makeup. It was great, except for one small thing: I had to watch myself on television. You see, for a girl like me, there are two problems with that. First, everyone looks heavier on screen. Second, most people who work in front of the camera are impossibly thin to begin with. It was like being dropped into an alternate universe where everyone's smaller but you're suddenly bigger. I was totally and completely unprepared for how I would feel having to watch myself all the time. You know that feeling when someone shows you a photo of yourself, or you catch a glimpse on home video, and you're horrified? *Is that what I really look like?* you think to yourself. Well, I had that moment every single day. So how did I deal? I didn't. I snapped, my newly buff demons strolling right back into my life.

Within three months of getting that job, I developed a raging eating disorder, descending into my darkest period. I should have been having the time of my life: twenty-two years old; living in New York; dream job; decent salary; great boyfriend. Nothing Aunt Shirley had predicted was true. Still, I dealt with my insecurities exactly as I had at nine years old, by bingeing. But this time, I wasn't sneaking a doughnut here and there. I would consume massive quantities of junk food—burgers, pizza, chips, cupcakes, and ice cream—*literally eating for hours*, until I went home and fell asleep. Then I would wake up and go right back out for more. I would wander the city and eat, like a zombie. Candy bar at the corner store. Eat it while walking to the deli. Ice cream sandwich at the deli. Eat it while walking to Burger King. Sit at Burger King and eat a burger, fries, and a shake. Walk to the pizza shop. Eat a slice at the shop and get one to go. Eat, rinse, repeat. For hours. Each and every day was filled with the desire to devour. It never went away. I would tell myself "not today," but the beast would say "just one," and they always won the argument. I felt utterly hopeless and powerless. And the worst part was watching it all unfold on camera, as I gained weight and started to look worse and worse. I was a wreck and everyone could see it.

Soon I descended into a full-blown depression. I was not well. If I wasn't working or eating, I was in bed, lights out, blinds drawn, even in the middle of the afternoon. I would lie there and pray for an accidental death, wishing I'd get hit by a car while crossing the street the next day, or some such fatal freak accident. I often fantasized about the mattress opening up and magically swallowing me whole. How lovely would it be to simply disappear?

Ask me how I climbed out of that hole and I have no clear answer. But by the grace of God, slowly, gradually, I did. Progress came in tiny increments. First, I stopped getting worse. I still binged regularly, but not as often, and when I did, the episodes weren't nearly as bad. They felt more like brief periods of release than a total and complete loss of control. The moments of deep despair became less frequent, until they virtually disappeared altogether. Then light started to creep in, and the greatest gift of all emerged: optimism. I got distracted by life—more interesting work, planning a wedding, renovating a home. I had things to look forward to. When I looked up, years had passed, and mercifully, I was okay. The darkness of my life gave way to dawn, then sunshine.

Looking back on that time, I realize one of the

worst parts of depression was that I had no idea how bad things were until I was on the other side. I didn't see how deep the hole was. Because of that, I now pay very close attention to my emotional state, always vigilant, like a night watchman. Making sure I'm feeling okay is a priority, because I never want the darkness to get a foothold again. What helps me the most with that is simply going through the motions. "Fake it until you make it," as they say. I still have days where something has gotten me down, and I don't want to get out of bed. But I go through the motions, one step at a time, and that always helps. Not sometimes, always. *Just get out of bed, Mara,* I think. *Just do that. Good girl. Now let's get dressed for the gym. You don't have to actually go. Just put your clothes on.* And so forth. The routine gets me through.

When it came to my body image after emerging from my depression, I was undoubtedly better, but far from fully healed. Thankfully, age and maturity brought a certain amount of acceptance and comfort in my skin, but I did in fact want to be thinner, to look and feel good. Furthermore, I wanted it to a permanent part of my lifestyle. I was exhausted from a lifetime of dieting and thinking about food. I wanted to be healthy, and more important, *sane.* So over the course of the next few years, I tried lots of different things to varying degrees of success. Of course I attempted every formal diet plan; counting points and carbs, signing up for programs online, buying weeks worth of prepackaged, vacuum-sealed food. At one point I even joined a bizarre food cult requiring members to adhere to absurd food restrictions, attend fellowship meetings, and completely submit to the direction of a more advanced "sponsor." While I did lose weight from time to time, nothing ever became a lifestyle. I always felt like I was sprinting through a marathon, which is completely unsustainable. At some point I'd stop running, and all of my progress would be undone.

After a time, I was done with all of the gimmicks. While part of me accepted a less than perfect reality, the desire to really live a healthy life was always present, like an old sports injury. You may move through life like everyone else, but you always feel that nagging pain. I lived a double life. On the one hand, I was mature enough to realize that life's too short for self-loathing. I appreciated and loved myself, curves included. It wasn't an act, either. I really felt fabulous most days. Not only was I holding my head high as I moved through life, but since I was one of the few plus-sized women on television, I also felt a tremendous sense of pride in representing the average woman with style and poise. I took that very seriously and wore it as a badge of honor. If I walked around like a shrinking violet, ashamed of my size, what did that say about our viewers, most of whom looked more like me than anyone on television? That's not me. I wore bright colors, the highest heel I could find, and hair so big and bouncy someone once asked me if I was from Texas, which I took as a compliment! But on the other hand, I still longed for the lifestyle I so desperately craved, one where I looked and felt as good as possible.

I ended up settling somewhere in the middle, between the years of radical dieting, and a miserable state of depressive binge eating. My default lifestyle became a genuine attempt to be healthy, but unknowingly going about it entirely the wrong way. I was working hard, but not smart. I ate virtually nothing but packaged food, things like frozen dinners and low-fat graham crackers. I wanted my food to be healthy, but effortless. I never cooked. I might as well have used my oven for shoe storage. If my meal wasn't packaged, it was takeout: a whole-wheat bagel at the deli, or a salad from a restaurant. I bought things that *sounded* healthy, like a slice of "yogurt loaf," which was essentially a big ol' piece of marble swirl cake. I genuinely wanted to do what was best for me, but I didn't know how.

Then there was the exercise part. Through the years, my fitness routine was as varied as my diet attempts. I went through a phase of working out to those cheesy TV fitness shows, the ones where people who look like they stepped off the set of a soap opera hop around on the beach. I went through a Tae-Bo phase, buying up anything Billy Blanks was selling. Every now and then I would jog, but I was always more excited about whatever cute gym outfit I was wearing than the actual workout. I absolutely hated exercising. I despised it. It was like going to the doctor: you know it's good for you, but it sure ain't fun.

Just like my diet plan, eventually my fitness routine settled into a default. While I did go to the gym, I thought I got points just for showing up. I didn't work very hard at all, most days reading *Us Weekly* on the elliptical for thirty minutes. If I wiped my brow it was just for effect, because I barely broke a sweat. Every once in a while I'd swing by some weight machine and do a few reps. Naturally, none of that gave me the results or consistency I was look-ing for.

Okay, so that's the sob story. Now to a happy place. Let's fast-forward to today. As I mentioned, I'm currently ninety pounds lighter than my heavi-est weight, and a size 6. It's the first time in my life I've been a single-digit size, and the smallest I've ever been. In fact, I often buy a size "small," which still boggles my mind. I always think to myself, *This must run big.* It's taking my brain a while to catch up.

For the most part, I have a great relationship with food. I eat fresh, healthy fare: mostly chicken, fish, eggs, fruits, veggies, and nuts. Generally speaking, I don't eat any flour, dairy, or grains, or drink wine (my beloved wine!). I cook 90 percent of what I eat: broiling fish, roasting chicken, and pureeing squash. I don't count anything. I don't measure portions. I'm not clocking the time until my diet ends. This is not a race. It's a well-paced walk through life.

I exercise every day. Not because I have to, but because I want to. I absolutely love my workouts. No, seriously. I love them. I'd happily get up from my computer right now to go for a run. Oftentimes working out is the most fun I'll have all day. I have endless energy, sometimes so much so that when I'm sitting in the office I feel fidgety, and start thinking to myself, *Man, I'd love to ditch this place for a workout.* As I mentioned, I used to go to the gym just to check a box. Now I go hard. I exercise intensely, whether it's Spin, running, or strength training. When I'm done, I'm drenched in sweat. If I'm not going to work hard, I tell myself, I might as well stay home. I leave the gym feeling empowered, energized, refreshed, and always wanting more.

My body has changed completely. Not just in the way I look, but in the way I *feel*. If I miss a workout or make a few unwise food choices, I *feel* it in a way that I never have before. It's like a hangover. I just feel totally "blech." My body is used to clean food and lots of activity, and when I don't get it, I feel lousy.

So why am I telling you all of this? Is it to flaunt my discipline and commitment to a healthy lifestyle? Hardly! I'm hoping that you find it comforting and inspirational. Chances are that no matter how long you've struggled with your weight or what kind of torture you've put yourself through, I've been there. There is no one less likely to succeed at a lifestyle overhaul than me. I'm not naturally thin. I didn't grow up playing sports. I love sweets so much I have literally poured sugar down my throat. But I did it, and you can, too. You absolutely can. Believing that has to be your first change.

If I'm honest, I also have to admit that I'm writing this for myself. Remember how in college I foolishly thought I'd won the weight war, once and for all? I'm much wiser now. I don't believe anyone vanquishes lifelong struggles. We all have our demons. Our best hope is to manage them. Given my history, it was really important for me to take note of my own personal journey, because I know for certain that at some point in the future I will need to refer to these lessons. I will never again be so arrogant as to believe that I'm cured. Unfortunately, Aunt Shirley lives in my head as much today as she did twenty-five years ago. I just do my best to keep her quiet.

Chapter II

THE FORMULA
Stumbling Upon Success

Before giving birth to my daughter, I had grand plans for losing the baby weight. I set up a little workout area in the basement and made an arrangement with my husband. He agreed to watch the as-yet born baby for half an hour every morning before he went to work so that I could exercise. I wanted to work out first thing in the morning, as a way to kick off each day of my maternity leave. In fact, I had an orderly and well-organized schedule for the entire day. If you're a parent, please stop laughing. I had no clue.

When the baby came it was like a tornado hit my house. I have never been so bewildered in my entire life, from the moment they put that gray, squirmy, gooey bundle of joy directly into my arms just seconds after birth (*You mean they don't clean her off first?!* I thought to myself). Having a newborn turned everything upside down. The house was a disaster, from dishes stacked in the sink to piles of laundry. Most days I would almost completely forget to shower or feed the dog. I was also breastfeeding, and my entire day revolved around creating food for my baby. I was literally feeding or pumping every ninety minutes, twenty-four hours a day, seven days a week. My life was reduced to one simple goal: make milk.

Needless to say, every single one of our plans went right out the window. Before my daughter was born, we decided not to use a pacifier. No binky for our baby! But within two hours of coming home from the hospital, that restriction went out the window, as we shoved bottle nipples into our daughter's mouth to keep her from screaming, until we could get to the store in the morning and raid the pacifier section. We'd decided against having her sleep in the bed; she needed to be in the bassinet. Well, she didn't end up in the bed, but she didn't sleep in the bassinet, either. Where, you might ask, did our precious baby girl slumber? In the only place where she would actually sleep: the car seat. That's right, the car seat, in the house, anytime she closed her eyes. We would just strap her in and carry it from room to room. We joked that she probably thought we traveled an awful lot, though we never actually left the house. And as for my well-laid fitness plans? Well, I exercised in the basement exactly once.

The problem was, I still needed to lose the baby weight. I'd gained forty pounds during my pregnancy, mostly due to an insatiable desire for salt. I ate macaroni and cheese like it was going out of style. I devoured ramen noodles several times a week. I put table salt on already salted potato chips. Extra salt on potato chips! Keep in mind, the forty pounds of baby weight were on top of the fact that I was already forty-five pounds overweight before my pregnancy. So after having the baby, I was the heaviest I'd ever been by far, and I didn't want to stay that way. But I also quickly realized that when it came to my life at that moment in time, there was no way I could do anything but tread water. Trying to get to the gym was simply too much, let alone summoning the energy to actually exercise. I was tethered to my baby via the boob. So I did the only thing I could. I focused solely on what I was eating. Right from the beginning, I made sure I was eating healthy foods in reasonable portions that I would prepare myself at home. (I'll detail specifically what dietary changes I made in the next few chapters.) Much to my surprise, by doing that alone, I lost all of the baby weight by the time I went back to work three months later. I'm not someone who has ever dropped weight effortlessly. In the past, every single ounce I've lost has been hard won. Yet there I was, forty pounds lighter from one simple and seemingly effortless modification to my lifestyle. This was a major breakthrough.

I could have stopped there, but I'd already changed my eating habits, so I thought, *Why not just keep going?* Four months later—seven months after my daughter was born—I was down another ten pounds for a grand total of fifty, all without ever stepping foot inside the gym. That's when I had my first and most important epiphany: *It's all about the food.*

As my daughter got older, my life settled into a routine, and I wanted to start exercising. I asked my friend Jenna Bush Hager about a Spinning class that she loved, called SoulCycle. She encouraged me to try it. So, one sunny Saturday in July I stepped into their Spin studio and clipped my feet into the bike. Let's just say the workout kicked my butt. The class is what you'd get if a regular Spin class had a baby with a wild night at the club, and then that baby drank a case of Red Bull. It is extremely intense cardio with great music, and some strength training and dancing thrown in. I left soaked in sweat. I mean, absolutely drenched. But it was a ton of fun. It didn't feel like a chore, the way most exercise always had for me. It felt like a party and went by in a flash. What's better than a fun workout? So instead of going to the gym, I became a SoulCycle junkie. I went as often as possible, up to four times a week.

You know how you have those times where you'll totally fall off track with your eating and exercise, and it just spirals down, getting worse and worse? One day off the wagon turns into a week, which turns into a month, and before you know it, your jeans no longer fit. It's a cycle many of us know all too well, especially me. But the good news, which I started to realize as I changed my life for the better, is that momentum works just as easily the other way. Once you get going, it starts to feel like rolling downhill, and that's exactly what began happening with me. The more I exercised, the more I *wanted* to exercise. As I started to get fit, I wanted to *be* more fit. It was a cycle of positive feedback. That's when I decided to start strength training and began going to another killer workout in New York called Barry's Bootcamp. Barry's is a combination of high-intensity sprints and incline runs on the treadmill and strength training with free weights. It's a lot like cross training, which is offered at many gyms. I thought I was in pretty good shape with all of the Spin I was doing, but this workout definitely humbled me! I barely made it through the first class, taking breaks repeatedly just to catch my breath. Lucky for me, also in the class were two fitness angels. Sascha Shutkind looks like she stepped out of a health magazine. The day I met Sascha she was wearing what she always does in class, nothing but a sports bra and biking shorts, and simply put, she was shredded. Arms, abs, legs, from head to toe, this woman was cut. Fortunately, she was as encouraging as she was fit. Even though we were complete strangers, she cheered me on the entire class. She pushed me to keep going. She congratulated me after every tough interval.

The other angel was the instructor. Noah Neiman looks like an action movie star: young, handsome, and ridiculously cut. Go do yourself a favor and Google "Noah Neiman shirtless." You're welcome.

Anyway, underneath Noah's granitelike exterior is a big ol' soft heart. Sure, he did his best to kill me during the class, but he did it with love, finding the perfect balance between pushing me to do better, and praising what I'd already done. Thanks to the two of them, I made it through, which goes to show just how important it is to surround yourself with the right people. That first class was grueling. I would even go so far as to call it torturous. But I left feeling ten feet tall, and just like with SoulCycle, I wanted to go back. I felt challenged, as though I'd just been presented with a new mountain to climb.

Sure, feeling good was great and all, but it didn't hurt that I started to notice results, beyond weight loss. I'd lost weight before, so getting smaller, while nice, wasn't novel. But for the first time in my entire life, I was becoming defined. You mean there were actually muscles under there? I would stand in front of my full-length mirror and flex like a bodybuilder, mouth open, stunned that I could actually see them. Is that a bicep? Are those abs? I couldn't believe my body was actually changing. I also noticed that I was growing in other ways. I could run faster, for longer. I could lift heavier weights. I could Spin at a higher resistance.

Working out started to become the best part of my day. I didn't feel complete without it. My husband had to convince me to take one day off each week so my body could rest. It was then that I realized how futile my workouts had been in my previous life, going through the motions and barely breaking a sweat. The exercise changed me as a person more than anything else. It changed my body's tone and definition. It vastly improved my mood, overall happiness, and general energy level. I never saw any of those benefits from my prior halfhearted days at the gym.

Epiphany number two: *Train hard or stay home.*

As I began exercising more, I wanted to eat in a way that supported my fitness goals. I no longer wanted to be thin; I wanted to be fit. There's a huge difference. I began reading everything I could find about fitness and nutrition. What should I eat before a workout for the most energy? What should I eat afterward? What should I eat to build muscle? How much protein did I need? I wanted to be smart. If I was going to work my butt off at Barry's Bootcamp and SoulCycle, I didn't want to blow it all on breakfast later. So I made some major dietary changes, cutting out pretty much all flour, dairy, and grains. I'm not saying that's for everyone, but it was something I wanted to try and when I did, I felt liberated. Okay, to be totally honest, the sense of liberation came after six weeks of white-knuckle suffering. I won't lie to you about that. Anyone who doubts the addictive properties of certain foods need only try to kick the habit to realize how real that is. Ditching flour was one of the hardest things I've ever done, but also one of the single most important. Don't worry, I'll detail just how I did it in the rest of the book.

With all of the nutritional changes, though, my life was suddenly much more complicated. I had a very restrictive diet, on top of working out six days a week, sometimes twice a day. Remember, I'm not some independently wealthy socialite with a chef and a trainer. I'm a working mom with a very demanding career. For me to make everything work, I had to have a plan. Every single day. So that's exactly what I did. I started planning.

Each and every single day I'd ask myself two questions: What am I going to eat? When am I going to exercise? Every Sunday I'd go online and order my groceries for the week (I'm a New Yorker, that's normal here). I'd plan my workout schedule for the week and sign up for classes days in advance. Every night I'd look in the fridge and mentally plan out what I would eat the following day, as well as when I'd cook it. I'd pack my exercise clothes for the next day, and often my work clothes, too, including my entire makeup kit, several brushes, combs, and a flatiron. When you work in television, there's no such thing as rolling into work. You must be camera-ready from the moment you hit the door. That meant packing a lot of stuff for the gym. Then there was laundry. I was washing sweaty sports bras and running tights and socks around the clock. This probably sounds like a lot of work. The bad news is that yes, it absolutely is a ton of work. The good news? It's become completely routine. While it took some thought and effort initially, now I don't even think about it. Packing my gym bag is a ritual, like brushing my teeth. Figuring out what I'm going to eat involves a ten-second scan of the refrigerator, and sometimes a pop into the freezer to pull something out for defrosting. Like I said, momentum works both ways. But I learned that when I didn't have a plan, everything would fall apart. I'd end up with a fried chicken wing in one hand and a powdered doughnut in the other, watching *Oprah's Next Chapter* on the couch after having skipped my SoulCycle class, thinking, "Wait a minute, how did this happen?!"

Epiphany number three: *Planning is key*.

The last piece of the equation is my favorite. In doing my research on fitness and nutrition, I kept coming across guidance on the importance of sleep. I continued to discount it, because it's something we all hear all the time, and who doesn't want more sleep? It's not like anyone says, "I'd really like to be exhausted all the time." But we do the best we can, right? Yet again, and again, fitness experts all said the same thing. Adequate sleep is crucial. So I decided to give it a shot and sleep as much as possible, guilt-free. When my daughter napped, I'd nap, dirty dishes be damned. If I had to be up for work insanely early (which in the television world is really, truly insanely early), I'd go to bed insanely early the night before, which in the summer often meant turning in while it was still daylight. I'd even duck out of social engagements so I could go home and sleep. Yes, I became that girl, even though I'd always been the one to shut down the joint. I've never met a party I didn't like! But I made rest a priority.

So how did it work out? Wow! Those fitness folks are really onto something. I noticed a difference immediately. I mean, it was instant. Besides all the science-y stuff your body does when you sleep, like rebuild and repair muscles (blah, blah, blah), the benefits were much simpler than that. When I was well rested, my workouts were better. I had tons more energy. I made better food choices. I had fewer cravings for carb and sugar-heavy foods. Most important, I was better able to cope with all of life's stresses, which would normally send me to the nearest pizza joint. Anxiety, irritation, long hours, someone's dumb remarks, none of that bothered me nearly as much. The best part? When something did really bother me, I'd handle it by going to sleep! What's better than that?! I knew that a nap would make me feel better.

At this point you probably think I'm a nut; the idea of napping during the day is crazy. Normal people don't have time to nap on a regular basis. I get it. Most days I couldn't, either. I'd do my best to soldier through until I could get to the nearest bed and collapse into it. But I knew that if I could just make it to bedtime, everything would be okay, and just *knowing* that sleep was the solution to whatever problem I was facing was a huge plus. In the past, I'd almost always turned to food for whatever was bothering me, often because I couldn't pinpoint the problem. Now I know exactly what it is. Most of the time, I'm simply tired. I began having the kind of internal conversations with myself that one would have with a child. "I know you're cranky. It's time for your nap. Are you ready for your nap?" Believe it or not, that self-talk really worked, precisely because I was tired. I was speaking to my true needs.

The other thing I realized about sleep is that when you look for the time and really make it a priority, you'll find it. It's amazing how much more time is in the day when you turn off the TV, log off Facebook, put off chores for another day, and go to sleep. A lot of us live by the "I'll sleep when I'm dead" mentality. We consider it a virtue to slog through the day with a minimal amount of rest, as though life is some test of exhaustion endurance. Many of us also feel guilty about sleeping too much, equating it with laziness. But that makes no more sense than thinking of breathing too much as being greedy. There's no such thing as breathing too much. You take what you need. Sleep should be no different.

Epiphany number four: *Sleep is a necessity, not an indulgence.*

So that, my friends, is how I stumbled upon what I now affectionately refer to as "the formula," knowledge that led to my losing ninety pounds, dropping six dress sizes, and being able to lift something heavier than a can of soup while working out. I never planned on changing my whole lifestyle, and even if I had, I certainly would have gone about it a different way. As I've mentioned, I'd spent years working hard to lose weight, but not being smart. I wanted to do the right thing but I didn't know how. I was putting my efforts into the wrong things, often giving 50 percent to food, 50 percent to exercise (and not doing either very well, incidentally), and 0 percent to planning or sleep. But now, armed with the right numbers, I was ready to change my lifestyle in ways I'd never dreamed possible, all thanks to the formula.

Mara's Magic Formula

70% Food
+ 10% Exercise
+ 10% Planning
+ 10% Sleep
_____

100% Weight Loss and Fabulosity

Take a moment to really focus on those numbers. Do they surprise you? They sure surprised me, and as I share the formula with others, I find they often have the same reaction. I mean, think about it, if you just focus on the food alone and getting enough sleep, you're 80 percent there. Add in a few minutes of thoughtful planning each day and you're 90 percent there. The battle is practically won. No wonder it felt effortless.

I'm not anti-exercise at all. In fact, it's quite the opposite. No one believes more strongly in the mental, physical, and spiritual benefits of a good workout than me. Plus, you'll never get those Michelle Obama arms without some time in the gym. But I think exercise needs to be put in the proper perspective, and most of us don't do that. We hear that for sustained weight loss, we should focus on diet and exercise, so we equalize them. But it's not DIET & EXERCISE; it's more like DIET & EXERCISE. Food is by far the bigger factor. So, let's start there.

Chapter III

IT'S ALL ABOUT THE FOOD
Great Bodies Are Made in the Kitchen, Not the Gym

A few years back, I went to Chicago for a weekend visit with one of my best girlfriends from college. She's what we in my circle affectionately refer to as my "ride or die chick": we ride together or we die together, but either way, we're stuck with each other. This beloved friend of mine also happens to be the kind of woman who would be easy to hate. She's bubbly, sweet, successful, has a killer closet, and oh yeah, she's drop-dead gorgeous and model thin.

Though we'd been friends for more than a decade at the time of my visit, I knew virtually nothing about my friend's diet or lifestyle. I had simply always assumed that she was so freakin' thin and perfect because of good genes. Lucky her. From the outside, her teeny tiny waist, and the ability to maintain it year after year, seemed effortless. She never spoke about any struggles with food and seemingly never gained a pound. I thought she just breezed through life enjoying her good genetic fortune. Until my trip.

I arrived on a weekday while my friend was at work, and after meeting up to grab her house key, I went back to her apartment alone to bum around for a few hours. At some point, of course, I got hungry. But when I went to the kitchen, there was absolutely no snack food, either in the fridge or the cabinets. No chips, no bread, no cookies, no juice, nada. Begrudgingly, I got dressed and went out for a meal. I guess I should have known something was up then.

When my friend got home from work that evening, we went out to dinner. For her meal, she ordered an appetizer, and nothing else. *Hmm*, I thought. *Maybe she had a big lunch.*

The next day was a Saturday, so we were together all day. Not only did she not eat a big lunch; she didn't eat much of anything at all. The first time I saw her put anything in her mouth was around noon, and it was a piece of rolled-up deli turkey. One slice.

Over the course of the weekend, I'd see the same behavior over and over again. Though I stayed with her for three days, the only time I saw her use the microwave was to heat up some hair wax (sorry, girl). Another night we met up with some of her coworkers for drinks and they ordered a bunch of appetizers, including little pizzas. She didn't touch a thing, except for when she pulled a teensy corner of cheese (just the cheese!) off one of the pizzas, savoring it with an "Mmmm." That very moment is when it hit me: She's so thin because she's very careful about what she eats. Duh.

I'm not suggesting we all need to *be that* diligent about counting calories. But what I learned from that weekend is something that should be painfully obvious, but unfortunately isn't: Those who don't overeat, aren't overweight. Period. It turns out that you can't have your cake and eat it, too. It doesn't matter how many trips to the gym you make: what you eat and how much of it you scarf down will determine whether or not you lose weight.

Surprisingly, conventional wisdom doesn't reflect this at all. For some reason, we've taken all of the factors that contribute to weight loss—food, cardio, strength training, sleep, drinking water, carbs, protein, you name it—and we've equalized them. We act as though they all make the same contribution toward our success. Worse still, many of us prioritize the wrong things, like putting all of our emphasis on cardio and nothing else. Think about it; how often do you hear someone who wants to drop some pounds say, "I really need to get back into the gym"? For some reason, we think it's possible to exercise our way out of a bad diet, when you can't. That bears repeating: *You will never exercise your way out of a bad diet.*

For years, I bought in to the myth that I could. I thought I could pretty much eat whatever I wanted as long as I exercised a little. I would drag myself to the gym, sometimes in the middle of the night, because I was convinced that I needed to exercise to lose weight. I did this *for years.* Yet there I was, twenty, thirty, forty pounds overweight, all the while. Meanwhile, we all know thin people who wouldn't know what a treadmill looked like if they tripped over it.

The only reason I eventually figured this out was by an accident of circumstance. As I mentioned earlier, after having my daughter I just knew it would be impossible to exercise for a while. I was really, really upset about that. Not because I loved exercise the way I do now, I actually loathed it. I was upset because I thought there was absolutely no way I'd lose the baby weight without working out. But I was desperate to get back to my pre-pregnancy size, and a little desperation goes a long way. I was forced to change the one thing that I could actually control, and that was the food. I took it really seriously, because I knew there was no margin for error. This was it. "Either get your eating together or stay this size forever," I'd tell myself. Much to my surprise (shock, actually), it worked! The weight started coming off, week after week. Seven months later, I was down fifty pounds, all before beginning any kind of exercise routine. *But weren't you breastfeeding?* you may be thinking. Yes, I was, but only for three months. My rate of weight loss didn't change at all in the four months between when I stopped breastfeeding and when I started working out. I know some people swear by it, but in my experience, breastfeeding didn't do squat to help me lose the weight. You know what did? Eating less and healthier.

Listen, exercise *is* really important. It has a zillion benefits beyond burning calories. No one believes that more than me. Don't worry, we'll get to the part where I tell you to stop being as lazy as I was and start sweating on a regular basis. But that comes later, as it should in your journey as well. When it comes to losing weight, the food is far, far more important.

Any trainer will tell you that. Great bodies are made in the kitchen, not the gym.

For one thing, most of us vastly overestimate how many calories we burn during a workout. I've come to hate the calorie counter on the treadmill for that very reason. For example, at Barry's Bootcamp, I'll feel like I'm killing myself during the running portion of class. I am not a runner and I don't like to run. Like I said, it's the only workout I love after the fact, not during. I do it for the payoff, not the joy of the moment. Anyway, I'll barely make it through the fifteen-minute run, panting like a dog in July, shirt completely soaked through. If you were to ask me how many calories I burned during that run, I'd guess about 400 to 500. It's hard work! Then I make the mistake of looking at the calorie counter before turning the treadmill off, and it will say something like "180 calories burned." One hundred and eighty measly calories! I could eat that in one single mouthful.

The truth is, it takes a lot to burn just one calorie. Thirty minutes of vigorous exercise might buy you three hundred calories. Think about how little that is, in the scheme of things. Exercise is not going to compensate for your three glasses of wine a night, or your morning bagel. It's a numbers game. You simply can't do enough exercise to compensate for regular bad food choices.

The other thing about exercise is that it makes you much hungrier. It's ridiculously easy to eat back what you've worked off. Three hundred calories spread out over the course of the day are a nibble here, and a nibble there. It's not a ton of food. Add to that the sense of entitlement we get after having worked out, and you have a recipe for disaster. You might allow yourself dessert one night, or an extra cocktail with dinner because you went to the gym that morning. Well, there goes your 300-calorie deficit. Now you're working your butt off just to maintain your weight. And that's assuming you've accurately gauged how many calories you've burned. If you're overestimating how much you're burning, then you might end up *gaining* weight. Like I said, it's a numbers game.

Here's the great thing about figuring out the food first. For one thing, when you focus on the food alone, you can focus on the food alone. Completely revamping your lifestyle all at once is really, really hard. In fact, it can be downright impossible. Yet that's what most of us attempt. From one day to the next, we expect to overhaul our diet, eat less, tolerate more hunger, drink a gallon of water, take all of our vitamins, start working out an hour each day, and oh yeah, only drink alcohol in moderation and be in bed by 9 P.M. Ha! No wonder so many of us fail. But if you only pay attention to the food for a period of time, you won't end up so overwhelmed. Trust me, it's enough work to plan your meals and resist your biggest temptations. That's a full-time job in and of itself. Giving yourself time to do that allows you to get comfortable with the single most important part of your new lifestyle. Once you're in a groove, you can add more.

The other great thing about dealing with nutrition alone is that you'll get a really good sense of your resting metabolic rate, or how many calories your body burns on its own, day to day. You don't need to worry about figuring out a number. It's actually much easier than that. Eat less. Did you lose weight that week? Great. Your body burns more than that amount of food. Not lose any weight? You need to eat even less. You will very quickly figure out roughly how much food you need to eat to lose weight. Once you add exercise, do your best to eat roughly the same amount, and you'll lose even more. You may need to add a snack here or there, because pre- and postworkout nutrition is super-important. But you'll already have a realistic idea of how much you should be eating day to day, and can adjust from there.

It really is that simple. Not *easy*, simple. I hear people all the time saying things like, "I don't know why I'm not losing any weight." Well, I know why. You're eating too much. I used to say that all the time. It wasn't an excuse. I truly didn't know why I wasn't losing, because I thought I was doing everything right. But now, knowing exactly what I need to eat to lose, gain, or maintain, I can tell you that I was eating way too much.

A quick word about the scale, our unfairly maligned friend. Friend?! Yes, the scale is our friend. Why? Because it's an extremely useful tool to help you figure out what's going on with your body. A lot of people are anti-scale. They seem to think it judges them. I assure you, there's no back room where the scales get together and gossip about how fat we are. *It's just a tool.* People will say, "I use a measuring tape," or "I just go by how my clothes fit." Great. Those are tools, too. But why shun another really effective one in the process? The reason a lot of people avoid the scale is that it's discouraging. Believe me, I know that all too well. But I've come to think of the number it gives me as *information*, no more, no less. The scale is giving me very important information about my body. I don't need to freak out over it.

I weigh myself every single day. In fact, I firmly believe that *the more you weigh, the less you'll weigh.* Get it? The reason I do that is for one, it takes all of the anxiety out of weighing myself. It's not a "thing." I don't have to mentally prepare for weigh-in day anymore. I step on the scale, I look at the number, and I go on with my day.

Weighing myself daily has also taught me a lot about general weight fluctuations. It's not uncommon for my weight to fluctuate two to three pounds from one day to the next. Two to three pounds! So when I see that the number is up three pounds, that doesn't mean I've gained weight. It means I need to pay attention to the number tomorrow and the day after, and try to get a sense of what's going on. Maybe I ate too much salt and I'm retaining water. Maybe I'm PMS-ing. Maybe I actually have gained weight and if I wasn't expecting it, I need to figure out why. That happened to me a while back. Nothing in my diet changed (or so I thought), but I didn't lose any weight for weeks. I started writing down everything I ate, so I could analyze it. Turns out, my peanut butter habit had gotten out of control! Remember those 180 calories I said I could eat in one mouthful? Well, it's most likely peanut butter. I love the stuff, and while it's a great snack, you can easily overdo it. I scaled back the PB and voilà, all was right in the world. I never would have been able to solve that problem without the help of my friend Mr. Scale.

The peanut butter investigation brings me back to the food. I'm not suggesting you wait seven months to hit the gym like I did. If you're already working out and you like it, I'm not suggesting you stop. What I am suggesting is that you give yourself a period of time to figure out the food. You need time to get into the habit of preparing healthy, light meals. You need time to grocery shop, and organize your kitchen. You need time to pack your lunch for the following day. You need time to get used to not eating all of the evil stuff you love. You need time to see how your food intake affects your weight. Give yourself permission to take the time you need to make a really important change. How much time depends on you. Maybe it's two weeks. Maybe it's two months. You'll know when you've hit a stride. But don't rush! This is your foundation. Don't build a house on sand. We're creating bedrock here.

Chapter IV

EAT OUTSIDE THE BOX
Ditching Cardboard and Cartons

It was a bright, sunny Saturday morning in Harlem, and I had just returned home from grocery shopping. My older cousin was visiting from Italy, and he stood chatting with me in the kitchen as I put my food away. Now, just a little bit of quick background on the lovely Italian way of life, or *la dolce vita*, as it's known ("the sweet life"). Being that my father is Italian, we spent a lot of time there growing up. And of course, that meant lots of wonderful meals. (I've included recipes for some of my favorite childhood Italian recipes at the end of the book.) But as rich and hearty as Italian food is, it's also remarkably simple and fresh. Most meals consist of pasta (of course), grilled seafood, fresh vegetables, lots of tomatoes, olive oil, garlic, peppers, and fresh fruit. It's not uncommon for Italian women to go to the grocery store several times a week, so that there are always fresh ingredients in the house. This is the lifestyle my cousin was accustomed to.

So anyway, there we were in the kitchen, me unloading groceries, my cousin just hanging out. I pulled a stack of boxes from a bag—about twenty frozen diet dinners—and stuck them in the freezer. I grabbed two six-packs of canned tomato juice and put them in the fridge. A few large cans of soup went into the cupboard. Then came the snacks: a box of instant oatmeal packets, tiny little containers of applesauce, and a carton of low-fat graham crackers. You can imagine how all of this looked to someone who had grown up in Italy. When I was done putting all of my food away my cousin looked at me incredulously.

"What?" I asked.

"Do you eat anything that doesn't come in a box?" he chuckled.

The answer, quite simply, was no.

For most of my adult life, I ate packaged food almost exclusively, either junk food during a binge, or "diet" food when I was being "good." My normal diet was virtually all reduced-calorie or reduced-fat. But within those parameters, it was all ultraprocessed, high-carb, high-sodium crap. I didn't even eat real vegetables. I hated salad (still do), so I got my "vegetables" from canned tomato juice. The only fresh thing I ever ate was fruit.

I thought those things were good for me, because they were "light," and advertised as being healthy. But in reality, my diet was completely devoid of actual nutrition, and I was never fully satisfied because the portions were always so small. It was also unhealthy for me mentally. What I was basically doing was substituting the junk food I really wanted to eat with the diet version. Since I couldn't very well eat cake for breakfast, I'd have a low-fat muffin. If I wanted cookies for a snack, I'd have low-fat graham crackers. When I wanted ice cream, I'd have frozen yogurt. I didn't change anything about my relationship with food. As a result, I was frustrated and unfulfilled around the clock, and never lost any weight.

I was also spectacularly lazy. I didn't want to invest any time whatsoever in the food I ate, other than actually going to the store to buy it. I didn't want to peel or chop anything, I most definitely didn't want to cook it, and the idea of packing a lunch seemed laughable. What I wanted was to pull something out of the fridge, microwave it, eat, and throw the container in the trash.

DETOX

Everything changed after I had my daughter. Because I had started focusing so closely on my food, it finally occurred to me that if I could purge my diet of those things I craved exclusively—carbs—then maybe, just maybe I could eat like human beings are supposed to eat. I took an honest inventory of all the things that were really a problem for me; those foods that I ate only to satisfy some vague emotional need, the ones I had no control over. These were the foods that I was chasing every moment of every day, often reluctantly cramming a diet substitute into their place. What would happen if I took them completely off the table? Would I be able to enjoy life without them?

Making that list required that I be totally and completely honest with myself. Because the only one I was accountable to was me, I could have easily been deceptive for the purpose of keeping treasured treats on the list. Not this time. I wasn't going to pretend that I could keep cookies around and eat them rationally, even if they were reduced-fat. Nope. Anything that had control over me had to go.

Here's what I came up with: all flour products, candy, and dairy. The dairy was only on the list because of ice cream, but I wanted to eliminate whole categories of food; going through individual items was too complicated and left me too much wiggle room. I needed black-and-white, no gray. I also added to the list white potatoes and all grains, because I quickly realized that I would have no problem substituting things like potato chips or caramel popcorn for the other stuff I was eliminating. I didn't want to substitute anymore. I'd been doing that for far too long. I wanted to see what would happen if I really and truly tried to detox.

After that honest assessment, this was my final list:

- All wheat flour products
- All dairy
- All candy
- All grains, including rice, couscous, cereal, and quinoa (though it's not technically a grain)
- White potatoes (sweet potatoes were okay)

I want to stress that this was *my* list. Yours may look completely different. If you can't control yourself around bacon, then that may have to go. Your list might even contain entire methods of cooking, if for example you have an issue with fried foods or baked goods. This is about eliminating the things you are abusing, because if you're anything like me, your food issues are likely built around those particular items.

After identifying what had to go, here is what I was left with:

Fruit, including:
Apples
Bananas
Berries
Peaches
Kiwi
Grapes
Cherries
Frozen fruit

Vegetables, including:
Broccoli
Green beans
Zucchini

Butternut squash

Spaghetti squash (a terrific substitute for
     pasta)

Asparagus

Eggplant

Mushrooms

Tomato

Avocado (yes, I know it's technically a fruit)

Spinach

Sweet potato

Animal protein, including:

Chicken

Duck

Cornish hen

Turkey

Salmon

Tilapia

Catfish

Shrimp

Tuna

Scallops

Lamb

I don't eat pork or beef.

Beans, including:
  Chickpeas
  Black beans

Nuts, including:
  Almonds
  Pecans
  Walnuts
  Pistachios
  Cashews
  Peanut butter
  Almond butter

Dairy substitutes, including:
  Soy milk
  Almond milk

Sugar substitutes, including:
  Splenda
  Honey
  Maple syrup

Though it looks long and plentiful now, at the time that list seemed pretty dire. I had no clue how I was going to get through it, but I was up for the challenge. I set a goal of forty days. I was going to abstain from everything on my list for forty days.

At first, my biggest challenge wasn't deprivation, but confusion. Stripped of everything I'd ever eaten, I had no clue where to start. In hindsight it amazes me that left with an abundance of *real* food, I felt like I had nothing to eat. When mealtime would approach, I'd draw a complete blank. You might as well have told me I could only eat foods that rhymed with "orange." I felt like I had zero options.

Slowly, though, I started to figure it out. Eggs and turkey bacon became my staple for breakfast. I intensely dislike cold, raw vegetables, so I started cooking them, and much to my surprise, they were really good! I'd sauté broccoli in garlic, olive oil, and lemon zest. I grilled mushrooms. I made a terrific tomato basil zucchini. It was all delicious. I discovered beans, which I'd never eaten before. They were a terrific and filling side dish. I'd cook black beans Spanish-style, or have falafel (made from chickpeas). For meat, I tapped into my love of seafood, eating shrimp, salmon, tilapia, and tuna often. I started cooking chicken a million ways. I learned how to make a mean roasted lamb! I even turned to vegetarian meat substitutes like veggie burgers because they were so easy to prepare. I also ate tons of fruit. One of the conveniences of packaged foods is how easy they are to grab and go. Not having those options was initially a challenge for me, but I found that fruit was just as easy to throw in my purse, and that's what I started to do.

I realized that if I was going to take the time to cook a dish, I might as well cook double or triple all at once, so I wouldn't have to cook as often. Before long my fridge was packed with storage containers full of a variety of different meats and veggies. Now, when mealtime came, I had too many options. I'd look in the fridge and marvel at all of my choices.

Okay, that's the uplifting part. But boy was there a downside. I can't lie about that. Letting go of the foods I loved was excruciating. I mourned a little bit at each and every meal, for weeks. I'm being totally serious. Every meal, I'd look at what I was eating and feel like I wanted to cry. Meals used to be fun and exciting. But these meals were boh-ring! All they did was nourish me. Ugh. That mental aspect was by far the hardest part. I expected my meals to entertain me. It was part of how I dealt with life. I had to get used to the disappointment of not having any food excitement at all, ever.

Changing my diet was literally the hardest thing

I've ever done. I felt like a smoker or drug addict going through withdrawal. I had headaches. I was irritable. I'd have cravings so terrible I felt like I wanted to punch a wall. It was absolutely awful. Often, the only way I got through it was by eating a lot of what I could eat. Being stuffed takes the edge off a little bit, even if it is from eating broccoli.

This is how a typical day looked during that time:

Breakfast:
    2 eggs, scrambled
    2 pieces turkey bacon

Midmorning snack:
    Handful of almonds
    Apple

Lunch:
    Large piece broiled salmon
    Broccoli
    Mushrooms

Midafternoon snack:
    No-carb snack bar
    Peanut butter

Dinner:
  Roasted chicken leg and thigh
  Asparagus
  Mashed sweet potato
  2 ounces vodka (in place of my nightly glass
    of wine)

Postdinner Snack:
  Apple
  Peanut butter

As you can see, that's a lot of food! Since this was detox, I did not limit myself on portions, log food, or keep track of calories as one would if it were a diet. My only single goal was to not eat foods on my banned list. Not surprisingly, I didn't really lose any weight during that time. But that didn't bother me, because as long as I was abstaining from certain foods, I was achieving my goal.

What really got me through those forty days were small goals. Most days, I didn't think about the full six weeks. I focused only on what was in front of me, and getting through that day, or sometimes that hour. I'd think, *Just make it to dinner. Just make it to dinner,* over and over, and drink a lot of water and eat some nuts, and before I knew it, dinner had arrived. Then I'd focus on making it to bedtime, and in the morning, I'd start all over.

Slowly, I got used to it. It was very, very slow. But once I started to feel "normal" again, it was even more motivation for me not to turn back. I didn't want to undo all of the hard work I'd done.

Once I hit the forty-day mark, I took a few days off, to eat whatever I wanted. I went for it all: pizza, chips, ice cream, doughnuts, cake, you name it. On the one hand it was fun, like being reunited with a bunch of old friends. But it was also remarkably disappointing. That food made me *feel* lousy: nauseous, sluggish, irritable, and bloated. It also wasn't nearly as good as I remembered. After almost six weeks of eating really high-quality, fresh food, for the first time ever I saw junk for exactly what it was. I could tell how low quality it was and how artificial it tasted. Everything was so much sweeter and saltier and fatty tasting than I remembered. Soda tasted like pure sugar, in a bad way. I remember not being able to finish a package of chips because they were just too damn salty. I was amazed by how much my taste buds had changed.

Not wanting to lose my momentum, after a few days of indulging I set a new goal of two weeks. After that I set another. And then another. Small goals have gotten me though the last two and a half years. I still set them. My current one is up in four days. When I get there I'll decide on the next one.

NEW REALITY

Today, I basically subscribe to a "clean" eating philosophy. My list hasn't changed much from when I first started more than two years ago. I don't eat flour, dairy, grains, white potato, or candy. I've also changed the way that I drink, cutting out wine. This was no small sacrifice. After all, as an Italian, I've been drinking wine since I was a child. Literally. I added wine to the list because that was completely undermining my weight loss efforts. I'm a very social person, and would regularly have friends over for a bottle (or two . . . or four). But it was making it impossible for me to lose weight. First of all, wine has lots of calories, averaging about 600 calories a bottle. Splitting one bottle with another person meant adding 300 additional calories to my day, and this happened several times a week. The calories you get from wine are also completely empty. It has virtually no nutritional value. You may as well drink a bottle of sugar. It had to go. I replaced the wine with straight liquor. That's right, straight, no mixers, no chasers. Now, liquor isn't any better for you nutritionally than wine; in fact, in many cases, it's worse, with vodka clocking in at about 60 calories an ounce, compared to 25 for wine. But I would never drink nearly as much straight vodka as I would wine. At the most I'll do two ounces, sipped slowly over the course of an hour or so, like an alcohol speed bump. It allows me to be social and relax a little, without completely undoing all of my hard work for the week. I realize that everyone can't drink straight liquor, so if that's too hard-core for you, feel free to add sensible mixers, like seltzer water or diet soda.

Getting back to the food, here's what I do eat: fruits, dried fruit (sparingly), nuts, vegetables, beans, chicken, and fish. I use soy milk and almond milk in place of dairy. The only grain I allow is corn, because so far, it hasn't become a problem. So if I really want to make something "breaded," I'll make cornflake crumbs in the food processor and use that. I use honey as a sweetener. If I really want a baked good, I'll make it myself, with almond flour.

Here's what I'll eat on a typical day:

Breakfast:
   Protein fruit smoothie (vanilla soy milk,
      vanilla protein powder, green tea extract,
      frozen fruit)

Snack:
   Apple
   Handful of raw almonds

Lunch:
   Broiled salmon filet
   Tomato basil zucchini
   2 baked falafel

Snack:
   Sliced grilled chicken

Dinner:
   Roasted chicken
   Mashed sweet potato with nutmeg, orange
      extract, and maple syrup
   Asparagus with olive oil

Dessert:
   Bowl of blackberries and blueberries, lightly
      drizzled with honey

Do I ever eat the things on my "banned" list? From time to time I'll make allowances for dairy, or a grain like rice, but it's almost always planned; something I've given myself permission to do. I've also found those things don't really have any power over me now, so I'm less cautious. The one thing I do try my very best to avoid at all costs is flour. It's the one thing that still (and probably always will) has complete control over me.

Do I ever fall? Absolutely. I'm far from perfect. Just because I set a goal doesn't mean I don't get some bumps and bruises on the way. And when I fall, I fall hard; often facedown into a pizza, spending days on a full-blown bender before I'm able to get back on track. It's something I remind myself of often; it's never just a taste, it's the beginning of a binge. That knowledge helps keep me on the straight and narrow.

The vast majority of the time, though, I manage to joyfully avoid my poisons, and to enjoy the abundance that is before me. It really is joyful, as all of my previous resentment and mourning is gone. I am free, and I am so very grateful for that.

My life before consisted of chasing my drug, my high. All I really wanted to do was eat. It's true. I would have been happy spending every waking moment eating baked goods, candy, and sweets. Because I wouldn't allow myself to do that, I lived in a constant state of discontent, always feeling deprived. Food was like a shackle. Now I feel completely free. Most times, most days, those things simply don't exist for me. They are not an option, so I don't think of them. My life is so much better now.

I feel much better physically. When I have a meal, I get nice and full; I'm not always in a partial state of hunger like before. I have tons of energy, and it's constant throughout the day, no longer dipping in the afternoon and other times. It's easier for me to wake up in the morning, and I have more energy when I exercise. I feel lighter, psychologically.

I'm also much lighter, physically! Perhaps the greatest thing about all of this is that once I eliminated my poisons, the weight loss became effortless. Truly effortless. Keep in mind, this is coming from someone who has had a lifetime struggle with weight. Virtually all of my excess calories had been coming from overeating very specific kinds of foods. Now that they're gone, I eat for energy, I eat to feel satisfied, and I'm not filling my body with a bunch of unnecessary stuff.

THE POWER OF HABIT

When you wake up in the morning, do you stop and think about the very first thing you'll do when your feet hit the ground? Do you lie in bed and ask yourself, "Should I go use the bathroom? Or should I eat breakfast? Should I brush my teeth or wash my face?" Chances are, you don't. The things you do every day, like brush your teeth or comb your hair, are habits. Your body does them on autopilot.

Habitual behaviors take place in a different part of the brain than the decision-making part. What that means is that you're not making a *decision* to perform so many of your behaviors each day. Think about how much effort it would take to *decide* to brush your teeth, or *decide* to tie your shoelaces. Your brain would be overloaded! Instead, habits help your brain work more efficiently, freeing it up for other things.

Researchers have found that the brain actually changes in response to habitual behavior. The patterns that we repeat most often literally become etched in our brain's pathways. Have you ever "zoned out" while making a cup of coffee in the same time, place, and manner you do every day? It's almost as though you look up and the cup just appeared. Or you pull into your driveway without having thought about the drive home at all. Habits also largely determine what and how we eat.

Part of the reason my dietary changes got easier over time was that my habits changed. Before, my autopilot was set to "unwise food decisions." Once I was able to hit the switch to "wise food decisions," my brain was suddenly working in my favor, instead of against me. While it's true that habits are extremely difficult to change, the good news is that you *can* change.

A habit has three parts: the trigger, the behavior, and the reward. So the first step in creating a new habit is recognizing the trigger. What leads to the habit? Is it arriving home after a stressful day? Is it finishing dinner and wanting something sweet? Identifying a trigger helps you figure out exactly how to replace the habit you're unhappy with. Specificity is key. Saying "I want to eat better" is very vague. Saying "I don't want to eat ice cream every night after dinner" helps you focus on a very specific habit.

Then you've got to determine what you are going to replace the bad habit with. *You must replace a bad habit with a good one.* Trying to simply stop a habit without filling it with something else is a recipe for failure. Remember, a reward follows the habit, which is why we do it in the first place. You need to figure out another way to get to that reward.

Now you're at the point where you want to *create* a new habit. The key here is repetition, and consistency. Repetition. Consistency. Repetition. Consistency. That's how habits are formed.

One way to create an environment for success is to make it as easy as possible to perform the new behavior. Even the tiniest obstacle can derail you, because remember, you're going against autopilot. For example, if you want to snack on grapes instead of chips, take the grapes out of the bag, wash them, and put them in a clear container on the top shelf of the fridge, right in front. Remove all possible barriers. Trust me, even then it will still be a challenge. You want to make the new behavior easy, and the old one more difficult.

One habit I wanted to change was mindless eating when I got home from work. I found that after getting home from a stressful day, all I would want to do is unwind. Even with my healthy eating in place, that often meant roaming the kitchen nibbling: a few grapes, some almonds, a piece of grilled chicken, a few forkfuls of mashed sweet potato, some peanut butter. It might seem like nothing, but it added up to several hundred calories every day. But that's not what bothered me. What bothered me about it is that I wasn't hungry at all. I was merely eating as a form of release. Relaxation was my reward. So I set out to change the habit.

I decided that my new habit would be to make a cup of chamomile tea the moment I got home. Chamomile tea has calming properties, so I figured it would address my real issue, which was the need to de-stress. Forming that new, extremely simple habit took a Herculean effort. I'd walk through the door and want to do a million other things before making the tea. But the longer I waited, the less likely that it was going to happen. I had to force myself to immediately make the tea after walking through the door. I'd even talk myself into it on the street was I was approaching home. "You're going to make tea, okay?" Eventually, it worked. Making the tea became natural. But it took time.

So just how long does it take to form a new habit? Well, it depends on how complicated it is. While conventional wisdom suggests it takes about three weeks, that's not always true.

One study asked ninety-six people to pick a behavior they wanted to turn into a habit, take note of how often they actually did it, and how natural it felt. Goals included things like eating a piece of fruit with lunch every day, or doing a daily fifteen-minute run.

After eighty-four days, researchers found that on average, it took sixty-six days for a habit to form. That's more than two months! But it wasn't the same for everyone. Those whose goals were easier, like drinking a glass of water after breakfast, formed a habit in as little as twenty days. Harder goals took longer to become habits, especially exercise-related ones. The study found that for some people, exercise still hadn't become a habit after the eighty-four days was up.

This shouldn't be discouraging. The good news is that at some point, the new habit will be formed. The harder the struggle, the bigger the gain. The important thing is to stick with it, repetitively and consistently.

Chapter V

FOOD ADDICTION
Twinkies Are My Crack

I remember the moment when I realized something wasn't right. I was twenty-two years old, and I was digging through layers of trash in my kitchen. Well, not really digging. I was actually lifting them up, so that I could hide the wrapper of an ice cream sandwich. I didn't want it to be right at the bottom, because then it could potentially show through the white plastic trash bag. Obviously, I didn't want it right on top, because then it wouldn't be hidden at all. No, it had to be just in the middle, surrounded by more respectable garbage. I nestled the wrapper in the middle of the heap, put a few layers of trash on top of it, and pushed down hard to smush it all together. And then I thought, *Wait a minute. Who am I hiding this from?* You see, I lived alone.

A short time later, I had another, similar experience. I was in the middle of a full-on binge, but out in public. At that particular moment I was in a video rental store, eating a delectable cake doughnut from Starbucks. As I rounded the corner, I saw someone I knew. I instantly recoiled, ducking *backward* into the aisle I'd just emerged from. *Oh my God*, I thought to myself. *What if she sees me eating this?* I peered through the aisles watching my friend peruse the shelves of DVDs. As soon as she turned her back I bolted out of the store. I was a full block away before reason kicked in. *Why would it matter if she saw you eating?* I thought to myself. *I mean, it's not like it's crack or anything.* Except, in my case, that's only partly true.

I know for certain, without any doubt, that I am addicted to certain foods. Aside from the eating in secret and the deep shame I feel about eating those foods, I also know that they make me high. I know this because I've spent a lot of time actually being high. Like so many young people, I experimented with a lot of drugs during my teen years, trying virtually every recreational drug available. Fortunately, though I danced with the devil, I never got burned. Nothing ever got out of control, my grades were always good, I finished college on time and went on to graduate school (on a full fellowship), and eventually, I just outgrew that phase. I was lucky. But I know what it's like to be high. And I know I get that from some foods. The euphoria. The profound sense of release. The irrational giddiness bordering on mania. And then an awful crash, punctuated by profound sadness, regret, and guilt.

Acknowledging this fact, accepting it, and modifying my behavior accordingly are the only things that have allowed me to make a significant change in my lifestyle. I am not on a diet. I am in recovery. An indulgence is so much more than a "slip"; it's a relapse. I also know that willpower is not the issue. No addict could be strong enough to have "just a little" of their drug. If they could, they wouldn't be an addict. Knowing these things keeps me tightly focused on why I've made these changes, and why it's so important to stick to them.

I know that I'm not addicted to all food. That would be terrible, indeed, because then I'd have to choose between addiction and starvation. No, I've never had the urge to binge on broccoli, or had to pour dishwashing soap over grilled chicken to stop myself from eating it. I've never eaten grapes until

I felt like my stomach was going to burst, and I've never had to plead with myself to please, please, please stop eating so many raw almonds.

I know exactly what my drug is: flour. Bread, cookies, cupcakes, doughnuts, pizza, pasta, waffles. You name it. Flour is my crack. I am powerless over it. It has reduced me to tears and prayer, often at the same time. As best as I can, so help me God, I stay away, and I know that this will be my reality for the rest of my life. I've mourned it, I've accepted it, I've moved forward. Does that mean I'll never eat flour again? No. I'm sure I'll relapse at some point. I'm not being fatalistic, just realistic. But when I do, I'll know that it's much more significant than "cheating" on a diet. It's a sign and a symptom of something much bigger going on with me, and I need to figure out what that is.

At the most basic level, there are three parts to addiction. First, you crave your drug of choice. Then you lose control over it. And finally, you continue using even though it's destroying your life. I can definitely check all three boxes when it comes to food. At my lowest I was "using" (that is, bingeing) all day, every day, even though it made me absolutely miserable and I wanted nothing more than to stop. I was powerless.

For years, the scientific community rejected the very idea of food addiction. Researchers looking for grants couldn't get any funding and were ridiculed by their peers. But over the last decade or so, a lot more research on food addiction has been published, providing evidence compelling enough that now, even the former secretary of health and human services, Kathleen Sebelius, acknowledges that for some, eating is "an addiction like smoking." There's good reason so many people are now convinced.

DOPAMINE

On the surface, the very idea of being addicted to food might seem implausible. After all, we need food to eat. Isn't that a little like saying you can become addicted to water? The answer lies in a lovely brain chemical called dopamine.

Dopamine basically makes us feel good. Really good. It is released in the brain's so-called pleasure center, or as I like to call it, party central. When we engage in something fun, like sex, or eating a yummy dinner, dopamine is released. This is the kind of manageable dopamine release your body can handle just fine.

When we do something super-duper fun, like drugs or high-stakes gambling, party central is *flooded* with dopamine, up to ten times what we get from sex. As you can imagine, that feels really, really good! We very quickly learn that this activity is the short-cut to fun times. Not only a shortcut, but in many cases an escape route as well. After all, what better way to beat the blues than a trip to party central? We start to seek out the dopamine-flooding activity as a way to feel good, *and* less bad when life doesn't go our way. Now we're hooked.

The problem is, those repeat floods of dopamine are a lot for party central to handle. Remember, the brain is equipped for booty calls and meat loaf, not heroin. So when party central gets out of control, the brain goes in and turns the volume down, *producing less dopamine or eliminating receptors altogether,* which means the poor addict has to use more of their drug to get the same effect. Trouble is, the user remembers just how great party central used to be, and keeps trying to get back there, even when it's not nearly as fun.

That's addiction, at its most basic level. You start

using a substance that floods the brain with feel-good dopamine, you love it, you do it over and over again, you get hooked, your brain chemistry changes, and then you're really screwed because now you're chasing a high you'll never reach again, and need more and more of the drug just to feel normal.

Of course, not everyone who engages in certain pleasurable activities will become addicted to them. I'm a testament to that. I have no lingering cravings or desires for any of the drugs I ever tried. Biology, genetics, environment, age, and several other factors will all play a role in who gets addicted to what, if anything.

For a very long time, psychologists and doctors thought only powerful drugs could cause addiction. But we now know that lots of pleasurable activities can hijack the brain, including food. This has been shown in many ways, including medical scans. One of the most significant of these studies found that the brain scans of obese people looked different than those of a normal weight. So just what set them apart? The brains of obese subjects lacked dopamine receptors. Party central had been shut down. Sound familiar?

In another famous study done at Yale in 2011,

researchers looked at the brains of twenty-six women who self-identified as food addicts (you can take a similar test later in the chapter). The researchers wanted to see if addictive eating and substance abuse looked the same in the brain. To do this, they hooked the women up to an MRI machine and showed them pictures of a chocolate milk shake. The women's brains responded by showing increased activity in the area responsible for addictive cravings, basically responding in the same way an addict anticipates a fix. They did the same test with women who didn't identify as food addicts, and they showed far less activity in those parts of the brain. They were not anticipating a fix.

Next, researchers let the women actually taste the shakes, because not doing so would just be cruel. Though the food addicts anticipated that sip far more than their non-food-addicted counterparts, when they actually tasted it, it was a big letdown. They showed less activity in the reward areas of the brain, which had apparently dulled over time. Just like addicts, they seemed to be chasing the idea of a great high, one that in reality was now unattainable.

The idea of using milk shakes for this study probably wasn't random. If the good folks at Yale had used carrots or grilled shrimp, they probably wouldn't have gotten such clear results. That's because not all foods are equally addictive. *What* you eat may play a very big role in food addiction as well.

PROCESSED FOODS

I don't know about you, but I've never heard of anyone being hooked on coca leaves. Sure, lots of people use them, mostly in South America, for everything from traditional healing to religious ceremonies. People chew them and cook them in tea, but no one is mugging their neighbors on the street to support their coca leaf habit. I have, on the other hand, heard of lots of people being addicted to crack cocaine, a force so powerful that it devastated entire communities across the country in the 1980s. So what's the difference? After all, they have essentially the same active ingredient.

The difference is, crack cocaine is a highly refined version of what's in the coca leaves. The leaves contain a very small concentration of the active ingredient in cocaine. It takes a lot of work to make a potent, expensive, powdery drug from shrubbery. First, the leaves are soaked in gasoline. More chemicals are added, and all of that is filtered through a cloth. The filtered substance is dried in the sun and then cooked in another chemical bath, leading to crystallization. Then the solvents are removed, and you have powder cocaine.

Crack is an even more refined version of the already-processed cocaine. It's made through a completely different process that consists of dissolving powder cocaine in water and baking soda, and cooking it until the crack separates out. So, as you can see, when it comes to coca leaves and crack, though you start with a relatively harmful natural ingredient found in a leaf, once you extract it, concentrate it, mix it with a bunch of chemicals, and process the hell out of it, you're left with something powerful enough to make mothers abandon their own babies.

Now let's take the same look at what happens to some of our food, like corn. While a lot of people certainly love corn, including me, somehow I doubt anyone has the urge to eat ten ears of the stuff in one sitting. That's because though it's sweet and delicious, all of the sugar in corn is packaged in good-for-you fiber and vitamins that slow its absorption. Plus, you have to work for it. It takes time to eat an ear of corn, and it leaves you nice and full.

High-fructose corn syrup is quite another thing.

First, dried corn kernels are soaked in sulfur water for a day or two. Then the middle part of the kernel, the germ, is removed, leaving behind a slurry of fiber, protein, and starch. Next, the fiber and protein and removed, leaving only the cornstarch. That's just the beginning. The cornstarch is mixed with hydrochloric acid and heated under pressure, breaking down the starch molecules and converting them into sugar. This syrup is then refined even more to remove water. This is corn syrup, comprised of dextrose sugar. But wait, there's more!

To make corn syrup into high-fructose corn syrup, you have to refine it even *more*, with various temperature, pressure, and acidity manipulations, converting the dextrose into fructose. This syrup is a supersweetener used in everything from soda, to salad dressing, to cereal. As you can see, high-fructose corn syrup has about as much in common with corn as crack does to a coca leaf.

The human body is built to deal with foods found in nature, like corn. Virtually everything natural that tastes sweet also includes fiber and vitamins. Nature never intended for us to strip all of the sugar from corn and sugarcane and toss all the nutritional stuff.

But we don't stop there. Once we've separated

the tasty from the nutritious, we combine these ele-
ments into amazingly tantalizing superfoods, like
sugary doughnuts and gooey milk shakes. High-fat,
high-sugar processed foods like these are a very recent
development, and our bodies have a hard time han-
dling them. Without any fiber or nutrients to slow
down their absorption, we get an immediate, intense
rush, triggering strong reward responses in the brain.
In terms of evolution, this makes perfect sense. The
brain wants to drive us toward high-calorie foods so
we can take advantage of them when we stumble
across them. This would have been really helpful for
our hunter-gatherer ancestors. The problem is, we're
not wandering around the plains looking for random
high-calorie foods to keep us from starving. In our
world, we have to work hard to *avoid* those things.

Certain combinations of fat, sugar, and salt are the
equivalent of food crack. They are blissful, melting in
your mouth and overstimulating the brain's reward
centers. They do nothing to satisfy hunger or provide
lasting, valuable energy. Our bodies were not made
to subsist on powerful combinations of concentrated,
refined foods, and these are the things that have been
shown to be most addictive. Chances are, the more

you stay away from processed, packaged foods, the greater your chances of breaking the habit.

These are some of the processed foods that used to be the foundation of my diet, but that I have now eliminated completely.

Breakfast Foods:
 English muffins
 Sliced bread
 Bagels
 Fruit yogurt
 Low-fat muffins
 Flavored oatmeal
 Sweetened cereal

Snacks:
 Graham crackers
 Rice cakes
 Sweetened applesauce
 Snack cups of sliced fruit in heavy syrup
 Microwave popcorn
 Crackers
 Frozen yogurt
 Chocolate spread

Lunch and Dinner:
   Precooked, frozen diet meals
   Pita bread
   Pasta
   Canned soup
   Sliced deli meats
   Cheese
   Jelly
   Tomato juice

Today, I try to avoid processed food as much as possible. I should note that processed isn't the same thing as "packaged." I frequently use packaged foods like grilled chicken breast and frozen fruit. But I look for whole foods in their natural state as often as possible. Many processed foods seem completely harmless, like rice cakes, for example. Sure, those things won't kill you, and they might not even make you fat, but my whole philosophy about food has changed. I want to eat things as close to their natural state as possible, just the way they arrived on this earth. The less it's been messed with, the better.

ANIMAL STUDIES

Several animal studies support the idea that food is addictive. First off, let me say that if you have to be a lab rat, a food addiction study is the one to get into.

Lab rats have been shown to like Oreo cookies better than rice cakes. No surprise there. They've been shown to like cocaine-infused water better than saline water. No surprise there, either. But researchers have found that they seem to like Oreos just as much as coke.

In this study, conducted at Connecticut College in 2013, researchers put rats in a maze with Oreo cookies on one side and rice cakes on the other. To no one's surprise, the rats spent a lot more time on the cookie side, eating chocolatey-cream confections to their heart's delight (by the way, they eat the creamy middle first, too). Then the researchers did a parallel experiment, putting liquid cocaine and morphine injections on one side of the maze, and saline injections on the other side. The rats spent more time on the cocaine side, because, apparently, they like to party.

What surprised researchers was that when they compared the two studies, the rats spent as much time on the Oreo cookie side of the maze as the cocaine side. When they measured stimulation, they found the rats' brains were *more* stimulated by Oreos than the cocaine, activating "significantly more neurons."

Another study wanted to answer the question of whether rats could become addicted to sugar. They tested this by offering rats daily sugar water, with about the same percentage of sugar found in the soda that you and I drink. When the rats were given the sugar water every now and again, they seemed to handle it just fine. But when allowed to drink it all the time, they started consuming more and more, while eating less and less of their rat pellet diet. Then the researchers took the sugar water away. Here's where it gets really interesting. When denied their sugar water, the rats showed signs of opiate drug withdrawal. Opiates, by the way, include morphine and heroin. Yes, the rats started behaving like drug addicts in withdrawal, exhibiting the shakes, chattering teeth, and higher anxiety. The shakes, people!

After a few weeks, the kindhearted researchers allowed their lab rats to have sugar water again. As you can imagine, those little furry guys were pretty happy to have their beloved sugar water back. So happy, in fact, that they pressed the release lever so furiously they consumed 23 percent more sugar water than they had before.

But by far the most interesting animal food addiction study I've come across involves binge-eating rats. In this case, researchers split rats into two groups. Both groups were offered delicious and fattening cafeteria-type food like bacon, sausage, chocolate, and cheesecake (I told you these rats were lucky). The difference is that one group got the tasty treats all day, and the other group only had access to them for one hour. Not surprisingly, the group with unlimited access to the fattening food overate and became obese. What's most interesting is what happened with the other group. When the yummy food came, they would binge on it. The rest of the day, they'd starve themselves, refusing to eat any of the healthy options provided to them! They were willing to wait for the good stuff.

The researchers then upped the ante. They added an electrical shock to the tasty food, so that the rats got a little sting when they'd eat. Would the experience of physical pain deter them from bingeing? Not at all, even when the healthy rat salad was shock-free.

WHAT DOES THIS HAVE TO DO WITH ME?

I don't believe that everyone who is overweight is a food addict. I also don't believe that all food addicts are overweight. (I'm sure there are plenty of thin ones walking around, too.) If you are, then hopefully, like me, you'll realize that recovery is the key to freedom, not another diet. But even if you're not, the evidence supporting food addiction is so strong that at the very least it points to the power food can have over us. If you're struggling with your weight, then I think it's helpful to realize what you're up against. Knowing your opponent is half the battle.

People frequently diminish the power of food, and the consequences of abusing it. While compulsive overeating may not kill you in one shot, like a heroin overdose, it can definitely catch up with you over time. It just takes a little longer than other drugs. We know that obesity can shorten life expectancy by as much as ten years. Think about how much time that is. Where were you ten years ago? What was your life like? What's changed since then? Now imagine all of it gone, simply because of food abuse. Even if over-

88

eating doesn't kill you, there's a very good chance it will affect your quality of life, as obesity has been tied to increased risk of heart disease, diabetes, some cancers, sleep apnea, and stroke. Then there's the psychological toll, feeling bad about yourself day after day, buying bigger pants and dresses year after year, getting more discouraged and depressed with each passing moment. The consequences of food addiction are very real.

My hope is that understanding that this is a very real problem, with very serious consequences, will help you fight the good fight, providing motivation to "stay clean." Part of the problem is that we've all bought into the nonsense that we're overweight because we "like to eat," or have poor willpower. But that's not the full story. Much of the reason we like to eat so much is that we're presented with the product of food engineering never before seen in the history of our species. Part of the reason we can't exercise willpower is that there have been real changes in our brain chemistry. Understanding the challenge helps you prepare for the fight.

SO . . . AM I A FOOD ADDICT?

If you really think you have a problem, you should talk to your doctor about it. But to give you a better idea of how food addiction is defined, here is the Yale Food Addiction Scale test.

YALE FOOD ADDICTION SCALE

The following question asks about your eating habits in the past year.

Answer options for this section:

0: Never

1: Once per month

2: 2–4 times per month

3: 2–3 times per week

4: 4+ times per week

In the Past 12 Months . . .

1. I find myself consuming certain foods even though I am no longer hungry.

2. I worry about cutting down on certain foods.

3. I feel sluggish or fatigued from overeating.

4. I have spent time dealing with negative feelings from overeating certain foods, instead of spending time in important activities such as time with family, friends, work, or recreation.

5. I have had physical withdrawal symptoms such as agitation and anxiety when I cut down on certain foods. (Do *not* include caffeinated drinks: coffee, tea, cola, energy drinks, etc.)

6. My behavior with respect to food and eating causes me significant distress.

7. Issues related to food and eating decrease my ability to function effectively (daily routine, job/school, social or family activities, health difficulties).

Answer Options for This Section:

Yes

No

1. I kept consuming the same types or amounts of food despite significant emotional and/or physical problems related to my eating.

2. Eating the same amount of food does not reduce negative emotions or increase pleasurable feelings the way it used to.

Scoring

A. For question 6 *or* question 7, did you answer "3" or "4"?

- ○ No—You do not meet the food addiction threshold

- ○ Yes—Continue

B. Is your answer the same as the response in bold, *for at least three of the following questions*:

1. I find myself consuming certain foods even though I am no longer hungry.
   (4)

2. I worry about cutting down on certain foods.
   (4)

3. I feel sluggish or fatigued from overeating.
   (3 OR 4)

4. I have spent time dealing with negative feelings from overeating certain foods, instead of spending time in important activities such as time with family, friends, work, or recreation.
   (3 OR 4)

5. I have had physical withdrawal symptoms such as agitation and anxiety when I cut down on certain foods. (Do *not* include caffeinated drinks: coffee, tea, cola, energy drinks, etc.)
   (3 OR 4)

92

6. I kept consuming the same types or amounts of food despite significant emotional and/or physical problems related to my eating.
   (YES)

7. Eating the same amount of food does not reduce negative emotions or increase pleasurable feelings the way it used to.
   (YES)

If you meet the food addiction threshold, you may want to consult a professional for further guidance.

Chapter VI

SLEEP
You Snooze, You Lose (Weight, That Is)

I've always had one master: sleep. More than anything else, more than food even, sleep has always had
complete control over me. For years, when my alarm
would go off in the morning, I'd ask myself one question: "Can I cancel whatever it is I'm getting up for?"
In college, the answer to that was almost always yes,
and getting class notes from friends quickly became
a substitute for actually attending my morning lec-
tures. I can still remember the horror of waking up
on the third day of my first week of real work after
graduating. The first two days were hard enough,
but on the third, I had the terrible realization that I
would not be able to cancel work, like, ever. I'd have
to wake up for it every single day!

Modestly speaking, I'm also very good at sleep.

Immodestly speaking, I would say I'm quite master-
ful at it. I can fall asleep anytime, anywhere. I could
curl up on the floor under my computer right now
and go to sleep. I never get jet-lagged, because when
it's time to sleep, even in a different time zone, I
simply lie down and drift off. One of my proudest
accomplishments comes from my talent for slumber.
I'm not sure if you're ready for this, ladies and gen-
tlemen, but I have actually outslept a cat. Yes, a cat.

The problem is, despite all of my talent for sleep,
I always fought it. I saw it as a curse, and not a gift. I
always felt guilty about sleeping. Why? Because society said that I should. Sleep equals laziness. Sleeping
too much is an indulgence. Naps are for toddlers and
Europeans. Going to bed early is for senior citizens
and boring, dull people. Conversely, sleeping little
is a badge of honor, and a mark of pride. You hear
folks humble-bragging about pulling all-nighters all
the time, proudly proclaiming, "I'll sleep when I'm
dead," and tweeting idiocies like "#TeamNoSleep," as
they power through another demanding day with a
cup of coffee strapped to their hand.

I know this mind-set all too well, because that
used to be me. Even knowing that I personally need
a ton of sleep, it wasn't a priority. I'd stay up as late

as humanly possible, sometimes until two or three in morning, and then schedule appointments early and all throughout the day. I too believed that it was a show of strength to drag myself out of bed and stumble through a long day, propped up by caffeine. Everything took precedence over sleep. It's not that it was low on my list of priorities; it wasn't even on the list!

Unfortunately, that misguided way of thinking seems to be more and more common. Most of us aren't sleeping enough, and that's increasingly becoming the norm. It's estimated that two in five people are sleep deprived, and that number has consistently gone up over the years. In 1960, the average person slept eight to nine hours a night. Think about it: without the Internet and dozens of cable channels, there's not a whole lot to do at night. In 1995, the average amount of sleep dropped to seven hours. Today, one-third of adults admit to sleeping less than six hours a night. As our amount of sleep has gone down, guess what's gone up? Rates of being overweight or obese. Sure, tons of factors influence the obesity epidemic. But sleep is a big one, and probably one of the least discussed.

I never set out to be a sleep advocate. Like I mentioned, I ignored my body for years. If the phone rang while I was asleep I'd quickly clear my throat before answering, and never, ever, under any circumstances admit I was asleep (come on, be honest, you've done that, too). What changed is that I saw the power of sleep firsthand, and that made me a believer. Let me explain.

While I was on maternity leave and trying to lose the baby weight, I came across a little piece of weight-loss advice related to sleep. It simply said that not sleeping enough could interfere with weight loss. I wasn't working at the time, and newborns do sleep an awful lot (though seemingly never at night), so I just started sleeping as much as possible. *I gave myself permission to do that.* Permission is key, because of all the guilt that's bundled up with sleep. I noticed a huge difference immediately. I wasn't as hungry. I wasn't craving junk food. I was in a much better mood overall, which helped me be at peace with the fact that no, I couldn't have macaroni and cheese for dinner every night. Months later, when I finally started working out, I noticed the amount of sleep I got made a huge difference in the quality of my exercise. For one, if I went to bed on time, I had no problem waking up for a 6 A.M. boot camp class. And the workout itself was much better; I felt full of energy, instead of dragging.

All of this taught me one very simple lesson: *Sleep is a necessity, not an indulgence.* Could I use all of that time spent in bed for something else? Sure. Is that something else more important than providing my body with a vital necessity? Unlikely. Now sleep isn't just on my list of priorities, it's at the very top. I have no guilt, and no shame!

Sleep deprivation is terrible on so many levels. Let us count the ways. Mentally, it makes it harder for you to focus, think through problems, and remember things. Insufficient sleep is linked to everything from car accidents to medical errors. Emotionally, it makes you more fragile, prone to temper tantrums and bursting into tears. Life's ups and downs are vastly magnified when you're running on fumes. Physically, it makes you sluggish, slow, and more likely to get sick. Being chronically sleep deprived is associated with a host of medical problems, including heart failure, stroke, high blood pressure, and depression. The Centers for Disease Control even calls insufficient sleep a public health epidemic. And, oh yeah, not sleeping enough makes it extra hard to lose weight.

One study even found that your degree of fat-ness is related to how little you sleep. They analyzed about one thousand volunteers who reported how much they slept each night. They found that those who slept less had more body fat, and that their percentage of body fat seemed to correlate with the amount of sleep they got. In other words, the less they slept, the fatter they were.

Let's take a quick look back at the formula, shall we? Sleep is 10 percent, the same amount as exercise. There's a very good reason for that. Studies have shown that not getting enough sleep makes you hungrier, more prone to eat junk like chips and pizza (no, seriously), and can even make you gain weight specifically in your belly (again, I'm totally serious). Sleep is the glue that holds all of the mental, physical, and emotional components together, so that you don't fall apart and right into a tub of ice cream.

SLEEP LESS, EAT MORE

A lot of really important science-y stuff happens while you're sleeping, so we should probably start there. I promise to keep this simple and painless. (After all, I'm the girl who failed the exact same chemistry class twice in college, convincing me I probably wasn't well suited for a career in medicine after all.)

The bottom line is that sleep is related to the release of several hormones that affect your weight. Some of them assist in weight loss and some contribute to weight gain. Ghrelin and leptin are two of those hormones. I like to think of them as the little devil and angel that sit on your shoulder. Ghrelin (pronounced kind of like "gremlin," appropriately enough) is the devil. Armed with a little red pitchfork, this hormone stimulates appetite. It's basically that evil voice inside your head chanting "Eat! Eat! Eat!" Leptin does the opposite. This kind angel sends a signal to your brain that you're full, telling you to stop eating.

Here's where sleep comes in. The amount of rest you get affects your body's levels of ghrelin and leptin, as shown in one study conducted by the University of Chicago. They took twelve healthy men, messed with their levels of sleep, and then measured ghrelin, leptin, appetite, and what kind of food they most craved.

Researchers subjected the men to two nights of sleep deprivation, where they were allowed four hours in bed. Then the men got two nights of extended sleep, allowed ten hours in bed. Compared to the nights of extended sleep, after being sleep deprived, ghrelin (the devil) was up 28 percent, and leptin (the angel) was down 18 percent. In other words, after only four hours of sleep, the devil on their shoulder suddenly became almost a third louder—practically shouting—while the angel got a fifth quieter, down to a whisper.

The logical conclusion would be that the men became hungrier, right? Well, that's exactly what happened. When researchers measured the subjects' appetites, they found they were 23 percent hungrier when they were sleep deprived. Imagine your appetite increasing by almost 25 percent, and then trying to eat *less than normal* in order to lose weight. Good luck with that.

The other simple truth is that when you sleep less, you're awake more, with more time to eat. I don't know about you, but I've never polished off a burger in my sleep. I have, however, eaten my fair share at 2 A.M. The longer you stay up, the more you're likely to eat, especially when that time is accompanied by an unusually large appetite.

BAD SLEEP = BAD FOOD

Have you ever noticed that when you're tired, you don't really feel like eating egg whites for breakfast? Or grilled fish for lunch? Of course you don't. For most of us, when we're exhausted, we go for comfort food, things like baked goods, fried foods, and sweets. There's a very good reason for that.

For one thing, it's called *comfort* food for a reason. It makes you feel good in the moment, with its delicious flavors and luscious textures. It may give you a quick and temporary high. And chances are, you have some personal association with that particular food. For example, my ultimate comfort food is a Twinkie. There's nothing better. When Hostess declared bankruptcy a few years back and Twinkie-pocalypse began, I went online and bought one hundred Twinkies. Yes, a hundred. Now, keep in mind that in general, I was eating one, maybe two Twinkies a year. This was a lifetime supply. But the thought of being Twinkie-deprived forever was just too much for me. Thankfully, the great Twinkie drought of 2012 was short-lived. But I digress. The reason I adore Twinkies so much is that my mother used to give them to me when I was little. Sure, she gave me lots of treats, but this one was my favorite, and we didn't keep them in the house. So from time to time, seemingly inexplicably, a Twinkie would appear in my mother's hand and I would go nuts. I feel the same way about them today. Comfort food brings us great comfort. Sleep deprivation is a state of discomfort. We humans don't like being uncomfortable. So one of the first ways we seek to ease the pain of exhaustion is through food.

Another thing we seek when we're sleepy is energy. One of the most common ways we seek supplemental energy is through caffeine. But we also look to food. For some strange reason, though, most people don't go for a nice plate of brown rice, sautéed broccoli, and roasted chicken, which would give us tons of energy. Nope. We turn to chocolate and soda.

Not surprisingly, when you're tired, you also have less willpower. Your body needs all of its energy to perform vital functions, and sadly, it doesn't consider resisting a snack to be one of them. You simply won't put up as much of a fight.

Remember the study of ghrelin and leptin? In that same study, researchers also took a look at what their sleep deprived (and hungrier) subjects craved the most. Turns out, their appetite for calorie-dense, sugar- and carb-heavy food like candy, cookies, bread, and pasta increased up to 45 percent when they were tired! Forty-five percent! The really fascinating thing is that their appetite for protein-rich foods like meat and nuts wasn't affected at all. Not exactly setting the table for wise food choices, now is it?

LESS SLEEP, MORE STRESS

Cortisol has been called "public enemy number one." You know a hormone is bad news when scientists start referring to it in the same way law enforcement talks about the mob.

Cortisol, commonly called "the stress hormone," is released in response to stress. In small doses, that can actually be a good thing, providing benefits like a quick burst of energy and higher tolerance for pain, in the event that you have to fight off a bear, let's say (or maybe just your boss).

Things get ugly when cortisol levels are too high for too long. If you're not able to get back down to your calm pre-bear-confrontation state, cortisol starts to wreak havoc, leading to things like higher blood pressure and lower immune responses.

Elevated levels of cortisol also have an impact on our weight, over time leading to loss of muscle mass, slower metabolism, and increased blood sugar, which in turn boosts appetite and a craving for sweets. As if that weren't bad enough, stress eating also tends to increase belly fat, exactly the spot where most of us don't want it. Aside from making that bikini especially hard to pull off, increased abdominal fat is linked to more health problems than fat found in other parts of the body, including higher risk of heart attack and stroke. It's also associated with higher levels of bad cholesterol (LDL) and lower levels of the good stuff (HDL). Increased levels of cortisol also make it harder for the body to burn fat for energy, which is exactly what we want it to do when trying to lose weight. Public enemy, indeed!

Here's where sleep comes in. Cortisol levels naturally rise and fall in the body throughout the day; they are highest in the morning and lowest at night. They dip before bedtime so we can get a restful night's sleep (imagine feeling ready for "fight or flight" just as you lay your head on the pillow; not exactly a recipe for calm shut-eye).

Sleep deprivation interferes with those natural fluctuations and leads to increased cortisol levels.

Less sleep means more cortisol, which means more of all the bad stuff we just went over.

Cortisol is particularly sneaky. It also interferes with your quality of sleep, creating the environment for a vicious cycle. You don't sleep enough, so your cortisol levels go up, which makes it harder for you to get good sleep the following night.

Much like the mob, cortisol is ruthless. It will slow your metabolism, make you want more sweets, give you a fat tummy, and make it harder for you to get good sleep when you do actually make it to bed. See why it's so important to keep it in check?

EMOTIONAL EATING

A few years back I secured an interview with General Colin Powell for a joint reporting project between *Ebony* magazine and MSNBC. In preparing for the interview, I downloaded a copy of General Powell's book *It Worked for Me* to my iPad. It's a collection of life lessons that guide him day-to-day. His very first rule was this: "It ain't as bad as you think. It will look better in the morning." He goes on to write, "A good night's rest and the passage of just eight hours will usually reduce the infection" (the "infection" being whatever ails you). At the time, this surprised me a little. Here was one of the country's most decorated and accomplished military men doling out his rules for life, and the very first one was about rest and perspective.

Now, of course, it makes perfect sense, because I've come to believe the same thing. Virtually any problem is improved with sleep, even just a nap. Nothing about the circumstances changes, but everything about your perspective does. A tragedy at night is a nuisance in the morning.

We know that sleep deprivation is linked to depression. But on a much simpler level, being tired just brings you down, decreasing your optimism and emotional resilience. All of this is intricately tied to emotional eating.

Most of us have engaged in emotional eating from time to time, if not on a regular basis. You have a bad day, a fight with your spouse, life just isn't going well, and you soothe yourself with food. For me, that used to be a part of my lifestyle. Almost every challenge was addressed with food. But now I've replaced that with sleep.

Knowing that sleep makes almost everything better, I have made that my number-one coping mechanism. That may sound awfully impractical, but it's actually not. I may not be able to sleep in that very moment, but I know that if I can just get to sleep soon, I'll be okay. That can mean taking a nap in a waiting room before an appointment, or deciding to sleep on a flight instead of staying awake to watch a movie. On days off it might mean taking a nap when my daughter does. Or it could mean going to bed absurdly early. If something's really bothering me, I figure, *Why stay up?* All it will do is give me more time to obsess about it and make it more likely that I'll reach for food to cope. When I wake up, I *always* feel better. Not sometimes. Always.

I've also learned that being tired is almost always *the reason* that I want to binge. Being a mom and watching the way my child interacts with the world has taught me that humans are generally pretty simple creatures. If our basic needs are met, we're happy. My daughter is cranky for two reasons alone: 1) She's tired. 2) She's hungry. When I'm feeling emotionally lousy and suddenly have the desire to binge, I ask myself, "Am I hungry?" If the answer is no, the next question is "Am I tired?" The answer is almost always yes. Tired leads to emotional, which leads to a binge. And it's proportional. The more exhausted I am, the more I want to eat. But it's so illogical. If I'm tired, the solution is to sleep, not eat. So that's what I try to do, as often as possible. Getting enough sleep helps keep emotional eating to a minimum.

THE DOMINO EFFECT

Like I mentioned earlier, sleep is the glue holding the rest of the pieces together. Remember, this life-style change thing requires a lot of work. Sure, it gets easier over time, but the tasks still have to get done. Those gym socks won't wash themselves.

Being tired makes you, well, tired. When you're tired, you don't go grocery shopping. When you don't have food in your house, you don't cook. When you don't cook you don't pack your lunch, and then you eat crap instead of nourishing, healthy food.

When you're tired, you sleep through your sched-uled morning workout. It wouldn't matter if you got up anyway, because you were too tired to pack your bag, and you don't have any clean sports bras because you didn't do your laundry. See what I'm getting at here? Sleep is the glue.

THE EXERCISE EFFECT

For a year recently, I worked the overnight shift. I anchored the first shows of the morning, from 5 A.M.

to 6 A.M. before filming for the *Today* show. As soon as I would get off work, no later than 8:30 A.M., I would go work out. Most days I'd make it to a 9:30 A.M. class.

Generally speaking, I was sleep deprived during that entire period. I didn't get great sleep during the day, because as it turns out, the world is a very noisy place in the middle of the afternoon. I'd often wake up intentionally in the afternoon to check email and communicate with "the land of the living." I was pretty much exhausted all of the time.

Yet and still, I made it a point to keep going to my morning workouts because it was the only time I could go. But let me tell you, they were just awful. I'd be dragging before the class even started. I was exhausted and didn't feel like being there. I just wanted to go to sleep. When I'd work out on weekends, after a normal night's sleep, I'd feel like Superwoman, full of energy and vigor.

As it turns out, my case wasn't unique. Studies have shown that being sleep deprived affects the quality of exercise. On top of that, researchers have found that when you're tired, you'll feel like you're exerting yourself really hard, when in reality you're not, so your results won't be as significant.

Not getting enough sleep will also affect your

results in another way. Sleep is when we get shredded. Adequate rest is key to building muscle, as that's when muscle tissue repairs itself and regrows. There's increased blood flow to your muscles when your body isn't moving, creating the perfect environment for muscle growth, and for men, human growth hormone reaches its peak during deep sleep.

HOW MUCH IS ENOUGH?

Seeing as how much time we've spent on discussing the "right" amount of sleep, at this point you may be wondering exactly how much sleep you need. That's a good question. The world's most sophisticated sleep researchers actually have a very complex method of determining if an individual is sleep deprived: They ask if they feel sleepy. Yep, that's it.

The amount and quality of your sleep is largely self-reported, and the only thing that truly matters is whether you feel adequately rested. Do you feel tired during the day? Do you yawn from time to time? If you were to get on an airplane, would you fall asleep? All of those things are signs of sleep deprivation. If you're getting enough sleep, you shouldn't feel tired.

Generally speaking, the amount of sleep one needs varies from person to person. Most adults need about seven to nine hours a night. Another way to determine how much sleep you need is to try a little experiment the next time you have a few days off. Go to sleep at a reasonable hour, don't set an alarm clock, and take note of what time you wake up. The first few nights, you'll likely binge sleep, especially if you're chronically sleep deprived. But after a few days, you'll start waking naturally after your body has gotten its rest. That will tell you how much sleep you need.

A lot of people are delusional about their sleep deprivation. Like I said, it's a badge of honor to sleep as little as possible and still function. A few years back, some researchers found a gene mutation shared by so-called short sleepers, people who genuinely need only about four hours of sleep a night. Once they made the discovery, they started a nationwide search for other short sleepers. They got responses from thousands who believed that they too possessed this gene, claiming they only needed a few hours of sleep a night. But out of those thousands, only a handful were legitimate short sleepers. The rest? Delusional.

If you need caffeine to help you get through the day, you're not getting enough sleep. Constantly relying on a drug to provide a state of alertness should not be the norm. Sure, it's extremely common, but it's not the way things are *supposed* to work. When you get enough sleep, you don't need anything to help you stay awake. You know what helps you stay awake? Sleep. Just because you can function well on little sleep and lots of caffeine doesn't mean your body is not paying the price. You might *feel* fine, but in ten years you'll have aged miserably and have a big, fat belly. So stop!

You cannot train yourself to need less sleep. Your sleep needs will gradually change over time (teens need a heck of a lot more sleep than senior citizens), but you can't condition your body to need less sleep at any given point in your life. The amount of sleep you need is genetically determined, and there ain't nothing you can do about it. If you consistently get less sleep than you need, you will be consistently sleep deprived, period.

BUT I DON'T HAVE THE TIME

The thing about sleep is that most people enjoy it, a lot. We fantasize about all of the rest we'll get on our next vacation. We binge sleep for twelve hours on the weekend. When the alarm goes off on Monday morning, we desperately wish we could just go back to sleep. So why is it hard to do more of something we all love?

Most people would say they'd love to sleep more, but simply don't have the time. There's so much to do, and only so many hours in the day. But that's just an excuse. If you make sleep a priority and look for more time, you'll find it. The reality is we waste a phenomenal amount of time each day. How much time do you spend watching TV, playing games on social media, shopping online, or talking on the phone? That's all time that you could be sleeping. It's a matter of sacrifice. If you make a commitment to sleeping more, even at the expense of things you enjoy, you'll find the time. The truth is, most things can wait, and a lot of others can be eliminated completely, because sleep is simply more important.

That being said, if you currently get six hours of sleep a night, no one's suggesting you immediately commit to nine. That's twenty-one more hours in one week. Sure, that would be ideal, but of course it's unrealistic. The goal should be to sleep *more*. If you're getting six, start aiming for seven. If you're getting seven, strive for seven and a half. Make sleep a priority and commit to getting more than you currently do.

The other thing to keep in mind is that your extra sleep doesn't have to be continuous. An eight-hour uninterrupted chunk would be best, but if you can close your office door and nap for thirty minutes instead of meeting a coworker for lunch, do it. If you can grab an hour-long "disco nap" before going out on a Saturday night, then you should.

Early in my career I spent years on the road chasing breaking news stories, which is always a hectic endeavor. You have an immovable deadline based on the time the show airs, regardless of what time zone you might happen to actually be in, and conditions are often challenging, to say the least. You spend all day running around getting information and interviews, logging tape, writing a script, and in my case, putting on fake eyelashes in preparation for a live shot. Depending on the story, this could go on for days, or weeks. So over the years, I developed a motto, which I still live by to this day: "Eat when you can, sleep when you can, pee when you can." It's all about immediately seizing opportunities to take what you need. When you see an opportunity to close your eyes for a few minutes, take it.

QUALITY SLEEP

Sleep isn't just about quantity. Quality is just as important. You can get all of the sleep in the world, but if it's bad, you still won't feel rested. Here are some tips for getting quantity *and* quality:

- **Easy on the caffeine.** Try not to drink caffeine for about five hours before bedtime. The effects linger longer than you might think. That includes things like chocolate, tea, and soda.
- **Limit booze before bed.** I know this seems counterintuitive, because passing out in a drunken stupor seems like a surefire way to get solid sleep. But researchers have actually found that while alcohol helps you fall asleep, it makes it harder to stay asleep and get quality sleep.
- **Create a tranquil sleep environment.** The bedroom should be used only for sleeping (and, ahem, maybe a few other things). If you use your room as an office and a playroom and your snack space, it can be difficult to unwind when it's time for actual sleep. Try to create a calm space that induces rest.

117

- **Black out.** Use dark blinds or curtains to keep out as much light as possible. Also, make sure you don't have a lot of blinking, flashing electronics around. All of this can disrupt sleep.

- **Disconnect.** Try not to engage with electronics directly before sleep. Studies have found that surfing the Web or playing on your phone before bed makes it harder to fall asleep. Give your brain some time to unplug and get ready for sleep.

- **Cool down.** My mother, God bless her, sleeps with the window open *all year round*. She says she needs fresh air, even in the dead of winter. It may be two degrees outside, but when you walk into her bedroom, the window is open, and she's a few feet away, bundled in pajamas and buried deep under a down comforter. Mom may take things a bit far, but it turns out she's on to something. The National Sleep Foundation recommends sleeping in a slightly cool room, around sixty-five degrees, as this helps regulate body temperature.

SLEEP DISORDERS

For some people, getting good sleep isn't a matter of will or priority. No matter how much they try, they have trouble falling asleep or staying asleep. Others will get a full night's rest and still wake up feeling exhausted. If this sounds like you, there's a chance you may have a sleep disorder. You owe it to yourself to get it checked out. Talk to your doctor about it, and if necessary, get a referral to a sleep specialist. Because if there's one thing we should all agree on by now, it's that getting enough quality sleep is important.

Chapter VII

FITNESS
Eat Clean, Train Dirty

Let me tell you a little bit more about how I used to "exercise." Though I've been overweight to some degree for most of my adult life, I have also always worked out. Two to four times a week, I'd drag myself to the gym, grudgingly. I absolutely hated to go. I'd think about it for hours beforehand, like a cloud was hanging over my head. It was a complete and total chore. Once I was there, I'd spend half an hour on the elliptical, or the stationary bike. I'd do my best to make the workout a little less tedious by reading a magazine or watching TV. At least then I could be entertained. If I was feeling ambitious, I might go to a random weight machine and do some reps, no rhyme or reason. I didn't even know what muscles they were working. The only running I did was out the door as soon as my thirty minutes were up.

Despite my halfhearted (aka "lazy") workouts, I really felt like they were beneficial. First of all, it took so much effort to get there that I felt as though I was making a supreme sacrifice, and surely that must burn some calories. I was also regularly "working out," so I thought I was getting all of the benefits, including a faster metabolism and a calorie deficit. I vastly overestimated how much of an impact my workout routine had on my life.

Today, my fitness life couldn't be more different. I exercise six days a week, first thing in the morning. This often means dragging myself out of bed before 7 A.M., even on weekends, even in the darkest, coldest days in winter. My workouts are intense. I run sprints and hills, I Spin like a madwoman. I strength train with free weights and resistance bands. I take ballet barre classes and yoga. I work hard and I leave completely soaked in sweat. But the biggest difference in my exercise routine then and now is that now, I love working out. It's the most fun I have every day. What gets me out of bed in the morning is that I'm going to do something really fun.

Up to this point, it may seem like I'm not a fan

of exercise. After all, I give it just 10 percent in the formula, and I've spent a lot of time talking about how insignificant it is compared to food. It's true that exercise needs to be put in the proper perspective, because so many of us overestimate its importance. But that doesn't mean it's not important.

Exercise is extremely important to overall health, in ways that go far beyond weight loss. In fact, I often remind myself that weight loss is the *least* significant reason to work out. Exercise is like a magic potion. It gives you lots of energy throughout the day and helps you sleep better at night. It not only prevents a ton of health problems like stroke and diabetes, but it also keeps you from getting sick in the first place by boosting the immune system. Best of all, it's been shown to improve your sex drive and slow aging. And, oh yeah, it makes you look great in a bathing suit.

As if that weren't enough, exercise is also really beneficial to mental health. It's a great stress reliever, it reduces anxiety, and some studies show it's as effective for treating depression as medication. Exercise also prompts the body to release endorphins, which are kind of like a natural version of morphine, providing a feeling of euphoria and reducing perceptions of pain. Happiness researchers (yes, such a thing exists) have found that exercise is one of the most reliable ways to boost overall life satisfaction.

I can personally vouch for these mood-boosting benefits. It doesn't matter how lousy or grumpy I feel, a tough workout always leaves me feeling happier, more optimistic, and energized. That runner's high actually does exist. I had no idea.

Since my fitness turnaround, I've seen tremendous results. I've already mentioned the weight lost—ninety pounds—but my body is completely different. For the first time ever in my entire life, I have some muscle definition. I'm nowhere near as shredded as I'd like to be (I'm getting there) but now I actually have *some* definition, whereas I used to have absolutely zero. I see it in my shoulders and back, my arms and abs, my thighs and my calves.

When I first started, I had no idea what I was doing. I really just wanted to start exercising to boost my weight loss. But it just so happened that I found a fitness class I loved, with SoulCycle. All of a sudden, I went because I wanted to, not because I had to. Those Spin studios were where I first fell in love with exercise. I was pushing myself for the first time, I was sweating like crazy, and afterward, I would feel so accomplished, strong, and energized that I wanted to do it again and again. Once I got hooked on exercise, I began seeking a fix wherever I could get it. I started doing Barry's Bootcamp and discovered a different kind of challenge. And so it went.

My goal today is no longer to be thin, but to be strong, and I've got to tell you, that's a much better way to live. Strong is not a destination, like a number on the scale; it's a journey. I'm much stronger today than when I started, and that makes me feel confident and accomplished. Yet I know I can be so much stronger, which motivates me day after day.

I have also discovered a whole new world of people, a group where working out every day and showing up to a 6 A.M. class in the dead of winter was normal. Changing my peer group had a massive effect on me, as it recalibrated my thinking. People who were more advanced pushed and encouraged me to work harder. We'd talk and share tips or challenges. I'd start meeting up with friends for a SoulCycle class and an egg white breakfast, not a pasta dinner and ten bottles of wine. Slowly, everything changed.

The more I changed, the more I wanted to change. I had tons of questions, like which foods would give me the most energy before a workout? Why was everyone with a great body so obsessed with protein? How often did I need to weight train? I started reading fitness magazines, blogs, and websites. I would ask my instructors specific questions after class. I found that knowledge is power, and that working smart was as important as working hard.

WORK SMART AND HARD

"Just get out there and go for a walk!" It's the kind of weight loss advice you hear all the time. "Take the stairs instead of the elevator." "Park your car farther away from the mall." They are small steps, we are told, that will add up to a big difference in reaching our fitness goals. Not so much.

If you get absolutely zero exercise, ever, then yes, adding any kind of movement is a good thing. It gets you used to more activity, and eases you into the idea of working out. If you have physical limitations like an injury, or you're recovering from surgery, then yes, you have to take it easy. But this kind of advice sets the bar far, far too low. This is precisely why I thought I should get a fitness medal for watching reality TV shows while riding the stationary bike.

If you really want to change your body, get lean and defined, build muscle, carve out a completely different shape, and have boundless energy, then you have to work *hard*. You need to push and challenge yourself every . . . single . . . time. An easy workout is a waste of time, time that you might as well use to sleep. When you're exercising, your heart should feel like it's beating out of your chest. You should be drenched in sweat. You should feel like you're lifting the heaviest possible weight that you can handle. Easy doesn't get results.

The key is to push yourself. You are *supposed* to be uncomfortable. The thing is, our bodies are very smart. Over time, they'll adapt to the stress we're subjecting them to, be it weight lifting or cardio, and it will become easier. As soon as it gets easy, you'll stop seeing results, because *hard is where the growth is*. You have to make sure that you're constantly raising the bar with more challenging exercises and heavier weight, so that your level of intensity stays the same.

When I first started exercising, the best I could do on a treadmill was a 4.5 mph jog, with no incline, a run that was really hard for me at the time. Today, I can run 7.0 mph, at a 7 percent incline, which feels just as hard. While I'm clearly in better shape, it *feels* the same to me, and it should. When 7.0 starts to feel comfortable, I'll move up to 7.5. As my friend, supertrainer Noah Neiman, says, "It never gets easier. You just get stronger."

Hard doesn't mean long. You should also be working smart, and that means you don't have to spend hours at the gym. You don't have to run ten miles. In fact, you shouldn't be working out for too long, because at a certain point your performance takes a dive. You'd be surprised how quickly you can get an intense, amazing, results-producing workout. If you work smart, *and* hard, 25–45 minutes four to five times a week will be enough. Your goal at the gym should be to get in, kill it, and get out. For most of us, that means unlearning everything we know about cardio.

Most people think that the way to burn fat and get into better shape is by doing the same exercise for a long time. For example, they'll decide to take up running, and run six miles at the same pace. That's called steady-state cardio, because you're not varying your intensity at all.

But new research shows that varying your intensity is actually much more effective. High-intensity interval training (HIIT) involves alternating between short bursts of high and low intensity. For example, on a treadmill, you might sprint as fast as you can for 45 seconds, and then recover with a light jog or a walk for 45 seconds. You repeat this for 25 minutes, 45 seconds on, 45 seconds off. The goal is to spike your heart rate at maximum intensity, and then bring it back down. The important thing is that your high-intensity intervals are actually high intensity. Intervals of jogging and walking are not going to be effective. During your high-intensity interval you should be running like someone is chasing you.

HIIT really is a gift from the fitness gods. Not only does it feel more manageable thanks to brief intervals, and give you a really great workout in a short amount of time, but it's also more effective than long periods of lower-intensity exercise, like jogging. You burn more total fat, and overall you're exercising at a higher intensity. HIIT has been shown to increase your aerobic capacity faster than traditional training, which means you'll be noticeably more fit much sooner. But best of all, HIIT gives you "afterburn," which is the fitness blessing of all blessings! After interval training, your body will continue to burn calories for up to twenty-four hours, while you go about your normal life. This does *not* happen with steady-state training. In short, you're getting a more effective workout in less time. How's that for a win-win?

Weight training is another way to work smart. Muscles burn more calories than fat, which means if you have more muscle mass, you're going to be burning more calories in general, even when you're doing absolutely nothing. Building muscle is a way to get your body to work in your favor, helping you to lose weight and be more efficient overall.

Just like with cardio, you have to work hard while strength training, or else you won't build muscle. Here's how your body builds muscle: When you lift a weight that's heavier than what your body is accustomed to, it tears and damages your muscle fibers. Later, your body repairs and rebuilds these fibers, and your muscle grows. But your body is good at adapting, and very soon it will be used to the weight you're lifting. The only way to build muscle is to submit your body to more stress than it's used to. The only way to do that is to lift progressively heavier weights. If the weight you're lifting feels easy, then you need to go heavier. You should go as heavy as you can without sacrificing form.

Ladies, don't buy into the myth that lifting heavy weights will make you bulky. That's nonsense. Women who look like bodybuilders work incredibly hard to get that physique. In many cases, that's their career, and they devote a tremendous amount of work and discipline into getting that body. Don't kid yourself and think you're going to look like that simply because you pick up a fifteen-pound weight. If only it were so easy!

Lifting heavy is another way to cut down your time at the gym. You don't need to do a million reps with a light weight. With a heavy weight, you can get great results by doing three sets of eight reps. Just make sure the weight is heavy enough that on that eighth rep, you really feel like you couldn't possibly do one more. Remember, it's smart *and* hard, not one or the other.

A quick note about working hard, for all of you overzealous readers out there—push yourself, but don't be dumb. The last thing you want is an injury, because that will take you out of commission for a while. You know yourself better than anyone. You know when you're being totally lazy and could do more. You also know when you're really pushing it and are likely to get hurt. Listening to your body is just as important as challenging it.

Your "mental game"—the way you think *during*

your workout—is going to be one of the most important factors. Your mind controls everything. Your body
is a slave. It will do what it's told. But you have to
tell it that you want to work hard, and you have to
mean it, even when your muscles are burning and
you feel like you can't breathe.

Everyone who works hard on physical improve-
ment has some mental trick they rely on. For me,
it's telling myself that the definition of strength is
pushing through the pain. When my body is screaming for me to stop making it so damn uncomfortable,
in that very moment, I think to myself, *If I can keep
going, despite this terrible feeling, I will be stronger than
when I walked through the door. Strength means pushing through the pain.*

I once asked Noah what he tells himself when
he trains. He said he thinks about the mechanics of
what he's doing, like simply breathing in and out,
or his form. "Focus on anything else but the pain."
Like I said, everyone has their tricks. Figure out what
motivates you *in the moment*. It's one thing to fantasize about wearing a bikini as you lie in bed at night,
but what's going to motivate you halfway through
a sprint when you can barely breathe? Figure it out,
because you'll need it.

DON'T RUIN IT WITH YOUR DIET

Watching what you eat is clearly a huge part of losing weight. But nutrition also plays a big part in getting in shape. As one of my boot camp instructors succinctly put it as I was leaving class recently, "Now don't go out there and eat a bunch of crap!"

One of the first things you'll notice when you start working hard is that you'll be hungrier, right after your workout, and all throughout the day. But to lose weight, or even just to maintain, you want to make sure you're not eating back all of the calories you've just burned off, which can be very easy to do. This is where you have to continue to work smart, scouring the universe for food champions that will keep you full and support your fitness goals without ruining your precious calorie deficit.

Naturally Low-Calorie
- This includes things like fruits, vegetables, lean meats, and whole grains.
- The key word here is *naturally*. Stay away from processed "low-calorie" stuff, as it's almost always full of empty calories and fillers that will make you hungrier in the long run.

NATURALLY LOW-CALORIE FOODS	
Food	Approximate Calories
Apple, medium	80
Blueberries, ½ cup	40
Romaine lettuce, 1 cup, shredded	10
Baby spinach, 1 cup	7
Asparagus, 1 spear	3
Shrimp, one jumbo	25
Chicken breast, one ounce	30

Fiber
- Fiber is your friend. The more fiber a food contains, the longer it will keep you full.
- Generally speaking, the harder something is to chew, the more fiber it has. This is not a scientific measure, by any means. It's just some helpful guidance.
- Great sources of fiber include most fruits, vegetables, and whole grains.
- Beans are an amazing source of fiber. One cup of black beans contains almost four times the fiber of an apple. Eat up!

HIGH-FIBER FOODS	
Food	Fiber (Grams)
Raspberries, 1 cup	8.0
Apple, with skin	4.5
Bran flakes, ¾ cup	5.0
Artichoke, cooked	10.0
Broccoli, 1 cup	5.0
Black Beans, 1 cup	16.0
Lentils, 1 cup cooked	15.0

Healthy Fats
- Fat is terrific at keeping you full.
- Don't worry about fat making you fat. Foods that naturally contain fat are almost always good for you, too. This includes things like avocado, nuts, and olive oil.
- Stay away from animal fat, as this is most definitely not considered a "healthy fat."

Protein
- Foods high in protein help to keep you full.
- Protein is really important for another reason:

135

It's the building block of muscle. Your body uses it to help repair all of those muscle fibers you've just damaged lifting weights. If you don't get enough protein, not only will your body be unable to build muscle, but it will eventually do the opposite, breaking down muscle to fuel itself, and you definitely don't want that. You can work your butt off in the gym, but if you don't give the body the fuel it needs, you won't see the results you want. It's quid pro quo: give your body what it wants, and it will return the favor.

HIGH-PROTEIN FOODS	
Food	Protein (grams)
Egg, medium	6
Chicken, 3 ounces	30
Salmon, 3 ounces	22
Steak, 3 ounces	19
Almonds, 1 ounce	6
Black beans, 1 cup	15
Soy milk, 1 cup	8

- The best way to get protein is to eat things like eggs, meat, fish, milk, nuts, beans, and soy.
- There's some debate about exactly how much protein you need. Some experts recommend one gram for every pound of your body weight. This can be a lot, though, especially if you're trying to lose weight. Supertrainer Noah recommends 20–30 grams per meal, which is very doable.

PRE- AND POST-WORKOUT NUTRITION

It's also really important to pay attention to what you eat before and after your workout. While we often use food for a number of different reasons, like entertainment and comfort, in reality, it's actually just fuel for your body. When you're getting ready to exercise, you'll want to give your body the right fuel for a killer workout.

Here's what experts recommend for your pre-workout snack:

- Eat about an hour before your workout.
- Don't eat too much, as you don't want your stomach to be too full.

- Aim for a snack, no more than about 200 calories, or a fistful of food.
- Try to eat a mix or carbs and protein. This can include an apple with a tablespoon of almond butter, a few ounces of grilled chicken breast and ¼ cup of brown rice, or half a peanut butter sandwich on whole wheat bread.

Even if you're on a low-carb diet, it's really important to eat a healthy carb before your workout. Your body *needs* carbs for energy. Think of them like gas for your car. Without gas, your car won't go. Without carbs, you won't physically be able to exert yourself for very long. You need them to power your workout.

Post-workout nutrition is also important, because you want to help your body recover as quickly as possible.

Here's what experts recommend for a post-workout snack:

- Eat within 15 minutes of completing your workout if possible, and absolutely, positively within one hour;
- Look for a mix of carb and protein, just like with your pre-workout snack.

JUST DO IT

When it comes to getting in better shape, one thing matters more than anything else. Without this, it doesn't matter if you work smart and hard. It won't matter if you exercise using high-intensity intervals. It won't matter if you lift heavy, or eat a perfectly balanced diet supporting your fitness goals.

The most important thing is this: consistency. Like the Nike slogan says, "Just do it."

Fitness gains aren't made all at once. They happen when you get a little bit stronger, day by day. It's like building a house. You lay one brick, then another, then another. But when it comes to fitness, you also lose gains quickly. If you don't build upon the progress you've made, it quickly disappears, and you'll never have that dream house. The only way to get stronger and more defined is to maintain what you've accomplished and build upon it.

The easiest way to make your workouts consistent is to find something that you really enjoy. It may sound like a cliché, but clichés exist for a reason. If you love your workout, it won't be such a struggle to get there. You may be thinking that it's impossible to actually love exercise. I used to feel the same way. I didn't understand how something physically uncomfortable could ever be fun. But now, I really do love my workouts, for different reasons. SoulCycle feels like a dance class, and I love to dance. Barry's Bootcamp isn't fun in the traditional sense of the word, but it makes me feel really strong and empowered, and gives me an endorphin rush that's amazing. I love them for different reasons, but what they have in common is that I love them. You have to really enjoy something if you're going to get out of bed at six thirty on a Saturday morning in the winter to go!

Getting there is 90 percent of the battle. If you torture yourself ahead of time by thinking about every grueling second, or how tired you are, you probably won't go. Don't allow your mind to go there. Tell yourself that your only obligation is to get dressed and go, and that if you don't feel like working out once you're there, you can go home. I promise that'll never happen. Gym clothes have magical properties, like a superhero's cape. Once you put them on, you'll be ready to fly.

Chapter VIII

PLANNING
Failure to Plan Is Planning to Fail

If you've ever been in a newsroom, you know that most of them are set up as big open areas, like a bull-pen, where producers and reporters can easily talk and share ideas. That also means that you can hear what everyone else is saying.

One day I overheard a conversation between a very high-profile war correspondent and a less-than-battle-tested entertainment reporter. The war guy had covered virtually every conflict of the last decade, often living in those areas for months on end. He has more lives than a cat. The entertainment reporter started asking him all kinds of questions about how he handles dangerous situations. Then she started telling him about all the self-defense techniques she knows. He listened patiently as she talked about all of the fighting classes she'd taken, and even gamely participated in a little demonstration.

"Here, try to hit me," she said, which he did, in slow motion, of course. She blocked it, and showed him a few other tricks. He never said a word. When it was all done, he finally spoke up.

"Can I tell you something?" he asked.

"Sure," she replied.

"If you're engaging in hand-to-hand combat, you're already fucked."

When it comes to the battle that we fight—the one with our weight—planning is the one thing that keeps you out of hand-to-hand combat. Because as my wise friend noted, by then you're already screwed.

There's definitely a huge emotional component to weight loss. For most of us, food is a lot more than just fuel. It's our comfort, our friend, and our little dose of daily excitement. In many cases it's also our drug. There's a lot wrapped up in how we eat, and some of it can be very tough to tackle. But a different set of obstacles are actually very easy to overcome if we simply plan.

An awful lot of our diet saboteurs have nothing to do with our emotions or our addictions. They have to do with laziness and carelessness. You set out to run a few hours' worth of errands and don't pack a single snack. You have a ridiculously busy day tomorrow and you don't go to bed on time or schedule an early workout. You show up at a holiday party ravenous, and then stand near the dessert table. You come home from work to an empty fridge. You give your husband's stash of ice cream top billing in the freezer, front and center, so it's the first thing you see every time you go for ice. Each one of those things could set you up for disaster and really get you off track. But the good news is, all of those problems are also easily solved. In fact, virtually every challenge can be overcome with good planning. You really *can* think your way through many of the toughest parts of weight loss.

Take a look at the Formula. Planning is 10 percent, the same percentage as exercise and sleep. Think about that. Planning is just as important as exercise and sleep. Depending on the circumstance, it may even be *more* important. Without it, everything else can fall apart. But planning isn't always easy, so I want to start with a few rules to help you get started. That's right, it's time to plan for your plan.

1. Suck It Up

I'll start with the tough love. The first rule of planning is to suck it up. Planning is a chore, plain and simple. Carrying out those plans is an even bigger chore. It's a full-time job. If it were easy, everyone would do it. Don't forget, laziness is probably what got you to this point; as in not cooking, eating out all of the time, never grocery shopping, skipping the gym. If you do more of the same, you'll get more of the same. Planning involves thinking through virtually every aspect of your life, including whom you are friends with. If you have friends who belittle your lifestyle changes ("Would it kill you to have one piece of bread? I mean, come on"), then they have to go. Planning affects everything. Accept that you're essentially taking on a new job.

Notice that I used the word *chore* above. That's essentially what planning involves: a new set of chores. Who wants more chores? No one! But if you want that tiny waist, you have to work for it, in more ways than in the gym. What if you don't like cooking? Too bad. Suck it up. You have to eat. You know what I don't like? Brushing my teeth. Seriously. I hate brushing my teeth. It's so boring; it just goes on and on. And then, as soon as morning comes, I have to brush them all over again. Despite all that, you know what I'd hate even more? Rotten teeth. So I do what I have to do, even though I don't like it. Our lives are full of obligations that we don't love but we do anyway. That's why they're called "obligations" and not "fun stuff."

2. No Excuses

Let's just stick with the tough-love part for a moment. Yes, I know your life is busy. Yes, I know you're juggling many responsibilities and maybe even kids, too. Yes, I know you barely make it through each day and don't see how you can possibly cram anything else into it. None of that matters. If you look for excuses, you will find them. As soon as you decide that you don't get an out, never, no matter what, you'll notice that you're resourceful in ways you never imagined. *It has to get done.* **The work required to support your lifestyle is not optional.**

Believe me, I get it. I don't have a limitless budget, a chef, a trainer, and endless free time. I'm a working mom who juggles a million things day to day, probably like many of you who are reading this. But most of your excuses are just that, excuses, not legitimate reasons to skip out on your plans.

There will be times when things fall apart. That's life. But they should be very few and very far between. As part of my job as a reporter, I've witnessed communities going through *real* obstacles, most often in the wake of a disaster. I've seen families go weeks without power or running water. I've witnessed others forced to sleep in tents or their cars. Sometimes their entire livelihood is on the line, as was the case with so many of the Louisiana fishermen I spent time with during the BP oil spill in 2010. *Those* are real challenges. But please don't tell me you had a bad meeting with your boss and that's why you stopped at the drive-through instead of cooking yourself a healthy dinner.

3. Know Thyself

The last rule of planning is to know thyself. It is really important to be honest about who you are, what you like and don't like, what your biggest strengths and weaknesses are, and what you are and aren't likely to do. Remember, the goal for all of this is success, and the best path toward success is to work with your nature, not against it.

If you really, truly despise cooking, how can you ease the pain? Can you devote a few hours on Sunday to preparing food for the entire week? Would buying a Crock-Pot help?

Are you really going to work out late at night after work? Really? Be honest with yourself. If work wipes you out and you're tired every night, that is not the time for a workout. On the other hand, if you're a night owl and look forward to a good stress reliever after a long day, then that might work for you.

Will you really wake up twenty minutes early to pack your gym bag and food for the day? Or will you hit snooze twice, eat up all of your extra time, and head out the door empty-handed? If you naturally wake up early and bum around reading the paper and sipping your morning tea, then great, do your packing in the morning. But if you're the type that's always running late and dashes out the door like your hair is on fire (like me), then don't kid yourself. Pack your bag at night so you can grab it and go.

Don't be afraid to tweak your strategy as you go. You may learn things about yourself that you didn't know, and will need to adjust accordingly. If you're consistently having a problem, just stop and *think* about it. If you always miss your planned morning workout, then maybe mornings aren't the best time for you (more on that in a minute). Maybe you can go at lunch instead. Or maybe you're not getting enough sleep and the problem would be easily solved if you went to bed an hour earlier. Just because something doesn't work right away doesn't mean you can't find the right solution eventually.

So what exactly does planning involve? At its most basic level, it means answering these three questions each and every day:

1. What am I going to eat?
2. When am I going to exercise?
3. When am I going to sleep?

FOOD PREP

Figuring out what you are going to eat will be the biggest component of your planning, as it should be, since food is by far the most important. Don't forget that. Don't pack your gym bag before you've made your lunch. Don't go to sleep if there are no groceries in your fridge. Food is your first priority.

When it comes to what you eat, leave nothing to chance. You never want to be in a situation where you have to figure out what you're going to eat at the moment that you're hungry. That's the equivalent of hand-to-hand combat.

1. **Groceries:** Do you have enough food on hand for the next few days? What are you running out of? When can you go grocery shopping? You will probably end up going to the store much more often than you do now, because when you realize you're running out of food, you must address it immediately. That may mean running out for a few odds and ends between big shopping trips.

Sample Grocery List
- ½ gallon light soy milk
- 1 bag frozen mixed berries
- Vanilla whey protein powder
- Carton of egg whites
- Carton of eggs
- Turkey bacon
- 8 apples
- 5 bananas
- 1 pound grapes
- 1 bunch asparagus
- 1 pound broccoli florets, in a microwave steamer bag

- 1 medium spaghetti squash
- Small bag of baby spinach
- 2 zucchini
- Minced garlic
- 2 small onions, pre-peeled and chopped
- Low-sodium chicken broth
- 2 salmon filets
- 2 pre-cooked skinless boneless chicken breasts
- 1 whole rotisserie chicken
- 1 pound jumbo steamed shrimp
- 1 bag raw almonds

2. **Cooking:** What are you going to eat for the day? When are you going to prepare it? Do you have all of the ingredients that you need? This is a daily process. I generally do it the night before. I'll pack my breakfast and my lunch, and do a quick scan of the fridge to make sure I have what I need for dinner. Preparing all of your food can be daunting at first, especially if you're not used to cooking. Here are some tips to help:

   ◦ A lot of grocery stores sell partly prepared food, things like diced onions, peeled garlic, chicken that's already been pounded thin, or green beans in a microwave steamer bag. Take advantage of that.

○ Buy frozen vegetables.

○ Cook much more than what you need and freeze part of it for later.

○ Buy much more food than you need and freeze raw ingredients. This will save you trips to the store.

○ Buy a slow cooker, such as a Crock-Pot. There's nothing easier than throwing a bunch of stuff into one pot and letting it do all the work during the day while you're gone.

○ Pack more than one meal at a time. You probably don't want to eat the same thing every day, but you can pack two of the exact same lunch, for example, one for Monday, one for Thursday.

3. **Packing:** What food do I need to take with me for the day? Do I need anything else to go along with it, like a plastic fork, or a wedge of lemon? Is the storage container clean? Will I have access to a microwave? Think through your entire food day and take what you need with you.

4. **Eating out:** Try to eat out as little as possible. You don't want to cede control of the single most important factor to someone else. Even things that look or sound healthy, often are not. This includes takeout and delivery. You want to prepare as much of what you eat as possible. That being said, life is about living, and we all go out from time to time. If possible, pick the restaurant yourself, so you can choose something that has all the options that you need. I'm a big fan of sushi, because a plate of sashimi is about as clean as food gets. I also really like steakhouses, because it's very easy to get a simple piece of grilled fish or chicken, with a side of steamed or sautéed vegetables. Just ask them to go easy on the butter. If you can't pick the place, take a look at the menu online first. You never want to see the menu for the first time when you're already hungry.

5. **Emergencies:** You should never be without an emergency snack. Things come up and you want to be able to go with the flow, not fall apart. If you planned to eat dinner at six and end up working

until eight, what are you going to eat to hold you over until you get home? Your emergency snack should be something nonperishable, like almonds or a snack bar.

EXERCISE

1. **Weekly plan:** Just as you should never grocery shop when you're hungry, you should never plan your workouts when you're tired.

   ○ You want to plan your entire week when you're alert and energized. Right *after* a good workout is a great time to do that, because you'll likely be really amped up and motivated. Remember, you want to push yourself and grow stronger, so don't plan easy workouts. Challenge yourself.

   ○ Planning the entire week allows you to make sure your exercise routine is balanced and well-rounded, that you're not overworking one body part and neglecting others, or getting too much cardio and not enough strength training. When you make a schedule for the entire week, you can really be sure you're covering all of your bases.

- ◦ If it helps, think of your weekly plan as aspirational. Stick to it as much as possible, but allow yourself the flexibility to accommodate life's ups and downs. The important thing is that you get your exercise in most days, no matter what. If that means going to an earlier class, or shifting things around a little, so be it.

2. **Early bird:** I am absolutely, positively *not* a morning person. I'm about as much of a night owl as one can possibly be, short of being a vampire. But I know that if I plan to exercise any time after noon, I more than likely won't make it. Working out first thing in the morning is the best strategy for success. As the day goes on, we all get more tired. Circumstances change, things come up, and before you know it's nine o'clock at night and you're exhausted. If you work out in the morning, there's less that can get in your way, you won't be worn out yet, *and* it will set the tone for the entire rest of the day, giving you energy and encouraging you to make better food choices.

3. **The gear:** If you exercise every day, you'll need a lot of workout clothes. Making sure you have clean clothes is part of your exercise planning.

- Once you've established a routine, I suggest buying at least one week's worth of tops, bottoms, and socks, so that you're not doing laundry every other day. This doesn't have to be expensive, top-of-the-line performance gear. Many discount retailers sell very cheap workout clothes. The only items that should be top quality are your shoes and your sports bra.

- Packing your bag: Stopping at home to change for the gym is the kiss of death! The comforts of home are too tempting. It takes a Herculean effort to come home, gaze at your comfy couch and your fuzzy slippers, and then leave it all behind to head back out into the cold, cruel world, to exercise, no less. You are much more likely to actually go the gym if you have everything you need with you. If your gym has lockers, even better.

SLEEP

Thankfully, this one is easy. You've already determined how much sleep you need. Now you must commit to getting it. This isn't complicated. It's about discipline and a devotion to giving your body what it needs.

For most of us, it's much easier to determine what time we go to sleep than the time we wake up. The time we get up is almost always determined by our obligations; otherwise, we'd stay in bed all day. So work backward, figure out what time you need to hit the sack, and then *do it*. Sleep sounds easy, but there's so much to do in life that it can be hard to get to bed. Going to sleep on time is actually very hard. It often involves either putting off something important, or interrupting something fun, like a great TV show. But you gotta do what you gotta do. Don't stay out late if you know you have to be up in the morning. Don't spend all night on the couch watching movies when you could be sleeping. Remember, sleep is the one thing that makes an instant difference. You feel it right away the next morning, and all through the day. Nutrition and exercise take much longer to pay off. Take comfort in knowing that you will thank yourself in the morning.

Chapter IX

FEEDING THE SPIRIT

I can do all things through He who strengthens me.

A few weeks after returning to work from maternity leave, I got an assignment for *The Today Show* which involved traveling to Washington DC. The story was about a pastor who held church in movie theaters. Being a new mom, I didn't want to be far from my baby—on a Sunday, no less. Frankly, I also wasn't very interested in the story. I didn't want to go, but I didn't have a good reason to turn it down. I agreed to do it.

I printed out my research and read it on the train to DC. The pastor's name was Mark Batterson. While reading his bio, I realized that he'd recently written a bestselling spiritual book, *The Circle Maker: Praying Circles Around Your Biggest Dreams and Greatest Fears.* I chided myself for not having realized this sooner, so I could get a copy. I like to know as much as possible about my interview subjects ahead of time, as it helps me understand them better.

When I arrived at the service, I realized the story I'd been assigned was kind of cool after all. The congregation met in a huge old movie theater. It was full of young people, all dressed completely casually, as though they actually were attending a movie. It was relaxed and welcoming. Much to my delight, there was a table in the lobby selling the pastor's book. I bought a copy to read on my trip home.

The pastor was a great guy. He was young and energetic, and came across as totally authentic and welcoming. I could see why his church was packed. When we were finished with the interview, I asked him if he would sign a copy of my book. He graciously agreed, writing "To Mara, Dream big. Pray hard." Thanks to his book, I would soon be able to do both.

I didn't grow up with any particular faith. My mother is Baptist, my father agnostic. We never went to church. I went to Catholic mass with my grandmother just once, and found it terribly boring. But I was always certain—always—that there was a God. I just had no clue how to get in touch with Him.

As luck would have it, when I got to college, my

assigned roommate was a super-devoted Christian. She read the Bible around the clock, even waking up at five in the morning to read and pray. She went to church twice a week. She was constantly befriending people and inviting them to church. So of course I used her as a resource. Who needs to read that big ole' Bible when your bunkmate already has the answers? I harassed her with questions *constantly*. Some were about Jesus, some about living a Christian lifestyle, others about heaven. I mean, this poor girl didn't have a moment of peace. But she patiently and lovingly answered every question I had, often opening the Bible to share a passage. Finally, after months of this torment, she looked at me and smiled the kind of exasperated smile a mother gives her child when they've just asked "why?" for the 500th time. "If you have so many questions about the Bible, Mara, why don't you just read it?" Good point.

I started reading the Bible, and along the way, I fell in love with God. Crazily, madly, head over heels in love. Most of what I knew about religion had been misperceptions based on stereotypes. This was nothing like that. It felt pure. I felt my spirit move within me for the very first time ever.

I found a church I adored, and started attending

every week. I would be so excited beforehand that I'd lay my clothes out the night before and go to bed early so that it would come sooner. Every Sunday was like Christmas.

Part of the reason my faith means so much to me is that I had to come to it on my own. I felt lost and without answers for so long that now I am tremendously grateful to have spiritual footing. But I am not perfect. I'm human. While most days my faith is strong, from time to time it gets tested. I'll be filled with questions that I can't find answers to, not in the Bible and not through prayer, and it's discouraging, causing me to wonder if God's promises are in fact real. That's the state of mind I was in when I began reading Pastor Mark's book.

One of the biggest struggles I was having at the time was about prayer. It had been in a spiritual conundrum for years. My issue was that I had already been blessed with so much in life that I felt guilty about praying for more. It seemed greedy and ungrateful. Of course, there were things I wanted in life, but I went about pursuing them on my own, which left me feeling guilty for not seeking God. I felt trapped. Couldn't move forward. Couldn't move back.

Three pages into Pastor Mark's book *The Circle Maker*, I was liberated.

> "Bold prayers honor God, and God honors bold prayers. God isn't offended by your biggest dreams or boldest prayers. He is offended by anything less."

He had me at hello.

I don't believe in coincidences. In this case that was more clear than ever. The whole reason for me being assigned this particular story was so I could read that particular book. God found a way to get me the answers I needed.

I devoured *The Circle Maker* in a matter of days, underlining passages as I went, writing notes in the back. It spoke to me on so many levels. One of them was on the concept of fasting. While the book is about prayer, it also makes the point that ". . . fasting is a form of praying hard." I had never thought of it that way. Pastor Mark goes on to write,

> "Fasting gives you more power to pray because it's an exercise in willpower. The physical discipline gives you the spiritual

discipline to pray through. An empty stomach leads to a full spirit. The tandem of prayer and fasting will give you the power and willpower to pray through until you experience a breakthrough."

After finishing the book, I was determined to put it into practice. Now feeling free to fully pray for what I wanted, I had to ask *myself* a question: *Well, what do you want?* Doing that was like opening up a floodgate. All of my privately held desires came pouring out. One of them was that I wanted to get my weight under control. Once and for all. I wanted to feel good about myself. I wanted to accomplish what I never had before. I wanted to vanquish my demons. It had always seemed impossible to me before. Now, I felt I had an avenue to get there: fasting and prayer.

Those first forty days without my poisons wasn't just a detox—it was also a spiritual fast. That's why I chose forty days; the same amount of time Jesus fasted in the desert. This was different than anything I'd done before. In the past, I'd prayed to God for help. This time, *I was making a vow.* The responsibility was mine. During that time I didn't touch any of my poisons *at all*. Not one morsel. Not one crumb. It was excruciating. It was beyond painful. The only thing that got me through was that vow. I didn't want to let God down.

Changing a lifestyle, overcoming an addiction, abstaining from one of the most powerful and constant forces in your life is remarkably, ridiculously hard. That's why so many of us have failed, time and time again. If you are a person of faith, draw on it in the face of this challenge. That's what faith is for, to sustain us through hardship. God wants you to be happy. He also wants you to be healthy. In fact, that's one of the most meaningful ways to honor the creation that is you. As I've gotten more fit, I've come to marvel at the human body and all it is capable of. This continues to be a spiritual journey for me. Every single time I begin an exercise—my first strokes on a bike, my initial steps on a treadmill—I silently thank God for allowing me to be there, moving without pain or injury, getting stronger, honoring His creation.

So what if you're not a person of faith? Are you destined to fail? Absolutely not. Everyone has some higher power. Everyone. Maybe you make a private vow to your children, promising to do everything you can to be there for them as long as possible. Maybe it's a vow to a deceased parent, saying, "Mamma, this is for you. I'm going to do better now." We *all* have something we hold sacred.

The power of faith isn't just crucial for changing your life—it's crucial for maintaining it. Everyone who has a problem with food uses it for a reason beyond hunger; it could be loneliness, disappointment, even boredom. If it didn't serve a purpose in your life, you wouldn't abuse it. If you're going to remove one powerful force, you have to replace it with another more powerful one. Caring for your spiritual self is an essential part of caring for the physical self. The two can't be separated. For example, there are plenty of spiritual conditions that manifest physically, like stress. Stress is essentially a disturbed peace of mind. That's a spiritual condition. But allow it to go unchecked and it becomes physical, tied to a number of illnesses. You must care for the spirit to care for the body.

My physical changes have been facilitated and accompanied by countless spiritual ones. This manifests itself in all kinds of ways, down to my breathing. Yes, breathing. One of the key things to manage during exercise is your breath. Whether my heart rate is on it's way up or slowly coming down, I'm monitoring my breath. In through the nose, out through the mouth, until I feel okay, settled into a new rhythm. Now, in life, I constantly do the same thing. When something is upsetting, I instinctively start to breathe. Deep breaths, in through the nose, out through the mouth, until I feel okay, settled into a new rhythm. I've started doing yoga for the sole purpose of lovingly caring for my mind and my body, stretching my muscles, slowing down my mind; physical and spiritual exercise in one. I do lots of other things that keep me spiritually fit, and have nothing to do with my physical self, from writing in a journal, to reading the Bible or a good novel, to just sitting quietly for a time. All of those things are about caring for my spiritual self. And they all keep me from the food.

I've come to believe that if God exists, so too does the devil. One can't be real and the other mythical. If there is black, there is white. If there is darkness, there is light. If there is good, there is evil. Several times now I've referred to my issues with food as demons, and I truly see them as such. They'd love nothing more than to suck me back into my former misery. The devil is a liar, and a convincing one at that. He tells me that I'll feel better if I give into those temptations. But I always feel worse.

The only way to drive out darkness is with light. Find your light. What truly lights up your life? Fill yourself with it, whether it's time with your kids or communing with nature on a hike. It doesn't matter what it is. Just find what speaks to your spirit and start that dialogue. Fight the demons. Don't believe their lies. The darkness isn't better. It's probably made you miserable for years. You will succeed. After all, you're not doing it alone.

Chapter X

OVERCOMING A STALL
A Setback Is Just a Setup for a Comeback

As I write this, I'm six pounds heavier than my lowest weight. It's three days after Thanksgiving, and I've spent the better part of the last week drinking wine and eating baked goods. Of course, I didn't plan to spend the week gorging myself, but I was hosting twenty people for the holiday and doing all of the cooking this year, and "one little taste" (to ensure the food was right for my guests, naturally) led to a daily eat-a-thon. I ate half a box of Nilla wafers while making banana pudding. I drank liqueur that I was using for cooking (one shot in the pot, one shot for me). I made a separate small serving of macaroni and cheese "for my daughter," but it went to Mommy instead. And this was all *before* Thanksgiving Day. While it reinforces my beliefs about the importance of staying away from my poisons, that's about the only silver lining. I'm so much worse for wear.

Now I feel physically disgusting: bloated, slug-gish, and nauseous. Thanksgiving night I woke up several times with a terrible stomachache. I'm always amazed at how the food I used to subsist on almost exclusively now makes me literally ill. Some things really are toxic for me and I need to stay away from them.

Mentally I don't feel great, either. I'm irritable, cranky, and really discouraged, feeling as though I've undone *all* of my progress. Of course that's nonsense. I know that you don't undo years of changes in just a few days. But it's easy to feel like a complete and utter failure, even if you've already accomplished a lot.

I'm sharing this because while I'd love to pretend that I'm a perfect model of change, that would be an outright lie. It's really important for me to share my struggles as well as my successes, so that you know you're not alone in yours. We all fall short of our goals from time to time, and that definitely includes me. I've had several setbacks since I started this journey, during holidays, birthdays, or just general moments of weakness.

Not all of my setbacks have been a failure of will. A few months ago I injured myself and couldn't work out for a few weeks. That wasn't my fault, but it was a major setback. In hindsight, it was no big deal. I don't think it cost me much progress at all. But at the time, I was devastated. As I've mentioned, my kick-ass classes are often the highlight of my day. Suddenly I was deprived of all my favorite activities, *and* my main coping mechanism for stress. That made things so much worse, because I was stressed and felt like I couldn't do anything about it. I was miserable and really worried I'd lose all of the fitness gains I'd made in stamina and strength. Of course, that didn't happen because, again, you don't undo two years of work in three weeks. But I still felt like a total failure.

In the past, I'd almost always respond to these kinds of setbacks by quitting. I'd be so discouraged and frustrated that I would essentially boycott all of my healthy changes, cutting off my nose to spite my face. *What's the point of doing all of this if I'm not making any progress?* I'd think. *Why am I working so hard for nothing?* Then I'd dig deeper into my rebellion by deliberately setting off on a binge. I'd decide I was going to enjoy all the things I'd been denying myself, because screw this dumb diet. I'd spend days eating whatever I wanted, and then get back to a more normalized kind of eating. But it would be months before I'd step back on the scale to assess the damage, or decide I was ready to give it another go.

In this new journey, I've had thoughts of quitting many times. It's easy to look at someone who has been successful at losing weight and think it's all linear, but it isn't. There are twists and turns, ups and down. I've set goals that have taken three times as long to accomplish as I'd planned, I've gained back a few pounds on several different occasions, and I've been extra-disciplined during certain periods only to step on the scale and be the exact same weight. So trust me, I know all about disappointment and frustration, even though overall I've done quite well. But what's different this time is that I never decided to quit. Not once. When I'm tempted to do that I always ask myself these questions: What does quitting mean? What are you going to go back to? Does that mean living a life of slavery to certain foods, as opposed to freedom from them? Does it mean feeling sluggish and unmotivated more often than not?

The life I'm living now is so much better for many reasons. Weight loss is just one of them. Even if I'm not losing weight or meeting my goals at the moment, I'm still much better off overall.

Setbacks are lousy. They are discouraging, demoralizing, and frustrating. They can be downright infuriating. I remember once being so angry that I hadn't lost weight after a particularly disciplined stretch, that I actually had to fight the urge to smash the scale. I'm not joking. I was going to pick it up and smash it against the wall. So trust me, I get it.

But here's the thing about setbacks: If you power through, they teach you how to make a comeback. It may sound strange, but the more practice you have with failure, the better you get at coping with it. At this point in my journey, having gone through setbacks time and again, I've realized that the important thing is persistence. Persistence is victory. All the clichés are true. It's not about falling down; it's about getting up. It's not about how many punches you can throw; it's about how many you can take. It's about having a healthy perspective, knowing that this is just a normal part of the process. Most important, it's about remembering that if you quit, you'll definitely never reach your goals. At least if you keep going, you'll get there eventually.

Still, getting back on track can be really hard. Once you've loosened the reins, it can be hard to tighten them again. If you've been eating cake and ice cream for breakfast three days straight (yes, I've done that), it can be tough to go back to egg whites. There's also a craving aspect to it. The less of certain things you eat, the less you crave them. But the reverse is also true. So if it seems like going back to clean eating is harder now, that's because it is. Your cravings have been reawakened. Then there's the emotional aspect, which is often the hardest to deal with. I always feel ashamed, guilty, sad, and angry with myself. Finding the motivation to start all over again can be harder than getting motivated on day one. That's a big reason so many people don't reach their goals. They fall down and just can't seem to get back up.

That being said, don't despair! Over time, I've found that the tools listed on the following pages help me get back to business right away. It doesn't matter if you're not very motivated at first; you likely won't be, given all of the obstacles detailed above. Just go through the motions, fake it till you make it, and in no time you'll be feeling stronger than before.

SURVEY THE DAMAGE

Facing consequences is tough, in all aspects of life, from finances, to relationships, to weight. It's much easier to stick your head in the sand than to look the truth in the eyes. Besides, when it comes to a weight setback, you're already feeling bad enough. Maybe your jeans are confirming your fears, squeezing you extra tightly these days. Why compound your misery with a great big number on the scale telling you just how much you screwed up?

When I've really been counterproductive—falling short of my nutritional goals, not making it to my workouts—I'd rather not face it. I keep telling myself that I'll confront the numbers *after* I've gotten back on track. The problem is, I find it absolutely impossible to get going again until I know exactly where I stand. Waiting only prolongs the process and leads me to fall further and further behind.

At the beginning of this chapter I mentioned that I'm six pounds heavier than I should be. How do I know that? Because I weighed myself this morning. I also took my measurements. It's not where I want to be. It sucks. I'm disappointed in myself. But this is the first step toward redemption.

Weighing yourself and taking your measurements are often the hardest parts of a relapse, because they force you to really confront the damage that you've done. At first that can be terribly demoralizing. I wish I could say that things are not as bad as they seem, but often they are, and sometimes they are worse. You might be horrified at the numbers staring back at you. But knowing them is one of the most important steps in picking yourself back up. Remember my mantra, "The more you weigh, the less you'll weigh." It's never truer than now.

Once you know where you stand, you can move forward with the other steps, detailed in this chapter. You probably won't want to do any more damage, so you'll curb whatever temptations you've been giving in to. You can set a new goal. You can also begin to let go of some of the guilt and shame, telling yourself. "Okay, I've gained such-and-such weight or inches. I'm not happy about that. But setbacks are part of the journey. It's time to move on now." Face reality, accept it, and move forward.

STOP DIGGING

What's the first step to getting out of a hole?
You stop digging.

Before diving right back into the deep end, you may want to give yourself a little buffer, if you will. This will be determined largely by your personality. Some people will only feel better by throwing themselves back into the game 100 percent. Others will feel so bruised and discouraged that they need a little more time. I've fallen into both categories, depending on the circumstances.

The important thing to do right away is not make things worse. No matter how bad it is now, it can always get worse. You should have some gratitude for wherever you are, even if it's not where you want to be.

For me, "stop digging" means doing the bare minimum, focusing on maintaining my weight, not losing. This could mean getting back to my dietary guidelines, but not worrying about portions just yet. It might mean a modified exercise schedule, or relying on more of my food substitutes than I should. It's basically a more relaxed approach that gives me a little bit of time to lick my wounds, regroup, and get back up. Sometimes it's based on logistical challenges, say if I'm traveling, or in the middle of the holidays. I try to do the best that I can until I can fully get going again.

NEW GOALS

Like I've said, baby steps have been the key to my success. I never set out to lose ninety pounds. I set out to lose five. Then five more, all the way down to ninety. Small goals are key. That's as true as ever when you've just had a setback. Once you've surveyed the damage and you know where you are, you can get back to the work of rebuilding.

Having a goal is the key to getting out of your stall and moving forward. It creates a mental shift. Now you're focused on the positive again, not the negative. You're looking forward, not backward. Hopefully, you have a new motivation.

It's important that your new goal be based on where you are *now*, not where you were before. If your goal is based on the past, it still forces you to look backward. Where you are now is your new reality, your new baseline, so build on that. Let's say you've gained thirteen pounds. If your goal "I want to get back to where I was," then after losing three pounds, you'll still be thinking, *I'm ten pounds from where I used to be*. But if your goal is to lose three pounds, when you've done that, you'll think, *Hooray for me!* and set the next one.

My new goal right now is to lose five pounds over the next two weeks. That may seem like a pretty aggressive goal, but knowing my body, I suspect I'm carrying a lot of water weight right now. Plus, I'm dying to dive right back in, so that number felt like a good way to get me motivated. It feels realistic and attainable, as long as I focus on what's worked before. Having a goal really helps get my head back in the game, and that's what counts.

SWEAT IT OUT

Sweat is like an instant reset button. It does wonders for the mind. I have found that absolutely nothing makes me feel better than a really tough workout. It makes me feel strong and empowered. It puts me in a better mood and gives me the healthy perspective I need. Most important, it starts that positive feedback loop. One good workout makes me want another one, and another one.

After a setback, I often don't feel like working out at all. If I've spent the last few days without exercising, a lot of my energy and motivation seems to evaporate. Plus, I often won't feel very sporty, with all the bloating and self-loathing going on. This is where my mind has to trump my emotions. I know with

100 percent certainty that a workout will make me feel better. I also know the first one back is always the hardest, so I might as well just go and get it over with. I force myself. I put on my gym clothes, I grab a banana and a pre-workout drink, and I just go. I always feel like a new person afterward.

BACK TO BASICS

Early on I mentioned that I wrote this book for me, so I wouldn't forget what steps had helped me change my life. I wanted to make sure I would always remember the basics so I could go back to them, because my old way of doing things continually tries to creep back into my life. That's why I remind myself often of exactly what works, so that I can keep doing it. It's all about the basics and that's never more important than during a setback. For example, I've stayed up way too late almost every night over the last week, ignoring my own rules about getting enough sleep. I know what you're thinking: *Oh, you rebel, you!* But in all seriousness, I know exactly what happens when I don't get enough rest. I don't get up for my workouts and I compound the problem by making bad food choices because I'm sleepy. So as I pick myself back up, I'm going back to basics. Tonight I will go to sleep

early. Before I go to bed, I'll pack my gym bag and figure out what I'm going to eat tomorrow. I've already
ordered my groceries for the week. I've gone back to
the formula, and the formula never fails.

The basics are the basics for a reason. They are the
building blocks for everything else. But because they
are so simple and elementary, we often assume that
once we've been doing them for a while, we'll never
need a refresher. That couldn't be further from the
truth. Old habits die very hard. In fact, I think they're
immortal. You can't kill those suckers off. They just
go hide and then try to creep back in again and again.
Keep those old habits at bay with the basics. Remind
yourself of what really worked in the first place, and
recommit to it. There's never a bad time to return to
your foundation.

MOVE FORWARD

What would happen if you drove a car while looking
only in the rearview mirror? You'd crash. You can't
move forward while you're looking backward. It's
something I've found to be true in many areas of my
life. For example, in my job, if I make a mistake on
live television, like stumbling or stuttering, I *cannot*
spend any time thinking about it, not one second, or

I'll just keep screwing up over and over again. Focusing on one mistake will only cause me to make several more. It's just as true in life. You must keep moving forward, or your past will destroy your present.

Recounting what you've done wrong is useless. If there's a way to learn from your mistakes, that's great, and it can be very instructive. But rehashing your shortcomings just to beat yourself up over and over again is pointless. Everyone falls. Get over it. Besides, what's the alternative? Be sad forever? Return to your old lifestyle? Of course not.

I have a saying: *The best way to move forward, is to move forward.* Just get up and look ahead of you, not backward. Don't think about how many slices of cake you ate. Don't dwell on all the exercise you didn't do. Don't count yesterday's calories. It's over and done. Forgive yourself and move on.

Chapter XI

FOR MY SISTAS

When I was in college I worked on a class project measuring body satisfaction among my peers. On a piece of paper, there were drawings of nine women's bodies (think a homicide chalk outline from *Law & Order*). The smallest drawing reflected the body of a woman who was underweight, the largest obese, the others incrementally in between. I handed these drawings out to about fifty of my female classmates, and asked them to circle two women: one reflecting the size they currently are, one reflecting the size they'd like to be. I also asked them to write their race on the page.

The results were fascinating. Every single white woman wanted to be smaller than they currently were, even when they were already underweight. But that wasn't the case with black women at all. While some certainly wanted to be smaller, others wanted to stay exactly the size they were, and some even wanted to be bigger!

When it comes to black women and our bodies, we have a certain confidence that lots of other groups don't have. It's reflected in so many aspects of our culture, from song lyrics ("Bootylicious," anyone?) to the black celebrities we look up to, who are almost always a little thicker and curvier than their nonblack counterparts. For black women, being bigger than the societal standard isn't only accepted; in many cases, it's desired. If only I had a nickel for every time I've heard a black person *insult* someone by calling them "skinny."

Research has found black women's self-esteem isn't necessarily tied to their weight. One study found black women who were overweight reported higher self-esteem and quality of life than white women of the same weight. This means they were more satisfied with things like their sex life and work. The study also found that when black women were worried about their weight, it was over their physical limitations, and not the mental or emotional aspects of being heavy.

That confidence was certainly true for me. When I was heavier, I never felt bad about myself. Sure, there were certainly times I wished I was smaller, mostly to be able to wear certain styles of clothing. But I didn't hate myself, or my body. I knew I was plus-sized, but I also knew I was fly. The two weren't mutually exclusive.

On some levels, I've always found black women's confidence to be in part a revolutionary act. You see, society rejects black women on so many levels, sending countless messages each and every day that our skin color, our hair, and our bodies are all wrong. Well, if the world is going to reject us anyway, then dammit, we'll embrace ourselves.

The confidence of my sistas is always something I have admired and loved. Life is too short for self-loathing. It's just not mentally healthy. Loving yourself, no matter where you are, is such an important part of life. Nobody should ever feel less-than. I think it's an attitude lots of others could learn from.

But there's a flip side to that confidence. It keeps us from talking about things that we should. Since we know we're fly, there's no reason to examine what might need to change. Why mess with something that's already fabulous?!

The truth is, self-love and self-improvement are perfect partners. You can't really seek to be better unless you truly care about yourself. While black women seem to be doing great on the mental health front, it's the physical part that's worrisome.

A few months back, I was moderating a panel at Essence Fest in New Orleans, a music festival thrown by *Essence* magazine, a lifestyle magazine for African-American women. All of the panelists were professional black women, one of them a doctor. As I always do before moderating, I asked each panelist if there was any particular topic they wanted to discuss. When I got to the doctor, she frowned a little, and nodded her head. "We have to talk about our weight," she said. "We don't want to talk about it, but we have to. It's killing us." Sadly, she was right.

THE STATS

Okay, okay, I know it seems like every other day another negative statistic about black women is released, as though researchers are just determined to tell us how dire our lives are. It's exhausting. I get it. But the statistics about black women and our weight are too important to ignore.

- African-American women have the highest rates of obesity in the country.
- 80 percent of black women over the age of twenty are overweight or obese. *Eighty percent.*
- For black women, the obesity epidemic cuts across socioeconomic lines and educational backgrounds, which is not true for other groups.
- Being overweight increases the likelihood of developing other health problems, including high blood pressure, diabetes, stroke, and heart disease.
- Heart disease is the leading cause of death for African-American women in the United States.
- African-American women are at greater risk for cardiovascular disease than any other ethnic group.
- 45 percent of black women have cardiovascular disease, compared to 32 percent of white women.
- The risk of heart disease and stroke increases with physical inactivity.

- Overall, 55 percent of blacks don't get the recommended amount of physical activity, compared to 44 percent of whites.
- 34 percent of black women are inactive, compared to 22 percent of white females.

One of the reasons I'd always discounted the statistics and guidelines about weight was that as a black woman, I felt they didn't apply to me. Something about those recommendations just didn't seem right. For my height, I am considered overweight at about 140 pounds, roughly a size 6. But in my community, a size 6 is generally considered average to small, and certainly not big. As a result, I discounted all of that information and decided to invent my own standards of what was healthy. I don't pretend to speak for all black women, which would be absurd. But I do know that a lot of us are doing the same thing. We're ignoring a lot of the information about our health because it feels like it doesn't apply to us. And you know what? In some ways that's correct.

There are lots of ways that black women are different when it comes to weight. Studies suggest that black women can be heavier than their white counterparts before their risk for associated health problems kicks in. In other words, our threshold for a healthier body mass index (BMI), and waist size, is higher. Plenty of research suggests we can be a little bit bigger and still be healthy.

There's also research to support the idea that black women are just a little bit bigger naturally. A recent study from the University of Pittsburgh School of Medicine found that black women may need to eat even fewer calories or burn more than their white sistas to lose the same amount of weight. That's right, when limiting calories the exact same amount and working out just as hard, the black women in the study were losing less. At first, investigators thought the black women might be cheating on their diets! But that didn't pan out. Then they looked at metabolic factors, but that didn't explain it, either. The end result was that after a six-month period, the black women in the study lost seven pounds fewer than the white women. So if you always suspected that junk in your trunk was a little more stubborn than your white girlfriends', you might have been right all along.

Then there's the issue of stress. All people of all races experience stress all the time, for all manner of reasons. But there's information to suggest that stress caused by racism is linked to weight gain. One of the ways racism affects its target is by creating a severe form of psychological stress. According to researchers at Boston University, black women who were the target of racist remarks and attitudes were at a higher risk of obesity. In their study, they evaluated 59,000 black women in 1997 and again in 2009, asking them how often they experienced racism like getting bad service at restaurants, or being discriminated against at work. Those who reported more experiences of racism were 69 percent more likely to become obese than those who didn't. This is one possible explanation for why among black women, being overweight or obese cuts across socioeconomic lines, which isn't true for other groups.

There are plenty of legitimate reasons why we tend to be a little bigger. But there's a big difference between giving ourselves a little wiggle room, to account for cultural and physical differences, and discounting all health guidance related to weight.

What I didn't realize all of those years was that in "setting my own standards," *I was actually cheating myself*. I saw a healthy diet and constant exercise as restrictive. I saw no upside, only sacrifice. And frankly, my community never challenged those ideas, because I was the norm, not the exception. Had I told a girlfriend I didn't want to work out because I just got my hair done, the response would have been "Yeah, girl, I get it," not "You can't be serious."

What I didn't know, and never heard discussed among my peers, was how amazing this lifestyle can be. By not challenging myself to change my diet and exercise habits, I was being cheated of so many benefits, from feeling energized all day, to being more optimistic overall, to getting noticeably stronger, physically and mentally.

I wanted to spend a little time talking just to my sistas, not to be preachy, but to share the gospel. I've seen the Promised Land, and it's beautiful. But with 80 percent of us overweight or obese, we don't hear that message often enough. We know that peer groups are extremely influential, so it's time we start moving our culture in a different direction. Not through nagging and judgment, but through *example*. If you're a black woman reading this, start with you. *Tell* people how great you feel, and *show* them how fantastic you look. Your commitment will be contagious, trust me. Your fellow sistas will see the Promised Land through you. After all, why should everyone else have all the fun?

Chapter XII

PARTING WISDOM

The truth is that I never set out to lose ninety pounds. Never in a million years would I have believed I could lose that much weight, nor that I needed to. I wanted to be smaller, but I had completely accepted that I would be "thick" or "curvy" my entire life. Thin was never part of the plan, and no one was more surprised by it than me.

The truth is that I didn't have a plan for success. I stumbled onto it, the way one finds a great new restaurant on a whim. I simply happened to try one thing that worked, then another, then another, and before I knew it, I had arrived at a destination I'd never set out for.

The truth is that once I made certain lifestyle changes, getting to that destination felt effortless.

Every pound wasn't a struggle. To the contrary, stepping on the scale became a pleasant and encouraging experience. I went about living my life and the weight just came off.

All of those things are the shiny, happy side of the truth. But there's also a side that's much harder to swallow. Brace yourself, because it's time for some medicine.

The key to everything I've said up to this point is that my journey felt effortless once I'd made certain changes. That's the good news. The bad news is that making those changes was hard. Excruciatingly hard.

Here's what's also true: they call it a lifestyle change for a reason. You have to change your life. Your entire life. *All of it.* That includes what time you wake up in the morning and go to sleep at night, what social engagements you accept or decline, even who you hang out with. If you have a friend who only wants to drink bottle after bottle of wine every time you're together, you might not want to spend as much time with that person. Everyone can't go on this journey with you. Sadly, some people will get left behind. Either they're with you, or they're not. On the other hand, if you have friends with a similar lifestyle approach, you can build around that, scheduling dates for a workout and healthy brunch afterward. If you're invited to three holiday parties in one week, you probably want to go to just one, or commit to staying at each one for less than an hour. No part of your life is unaffected. When you talk to people who are really focused on their health and fitness, you quickly notice that they build their whole life around those goals, not the other way around. It's a full-time job. Over time it does become as effortless as the lifestyle you're leading now. But please know that we're not talking about minor tweaks here. We're talking about a complete overhaul. Think about it: If you keep doing what you've always done, you'll keep getting what you've always gotten. If you want something different, you have to do something different.

It takes longer than you might expect for your new lifestyle to take hold. Like I've mentioned, I'd always heard it takes about three weeks to form a new habit, so when I first started making changes, that's what I was expecting. I girded myself for three tough weeks. But much to my dismay, it took about six weeks before I stopped feeling deprived and empty. While six weeks isn't a very long time in the scheme of things, it's a heck of a long time to go through withdrawal. It sucked.

Being adequately prepared for these challenges is crucial to success. In January 2009, my husband and some of our friends decided we wanted to attend the presidential inauguration of Barack Obama. I was told that I didn't have to cover it for work, which under normal circumstances would bum me out, but in this case was just fine by me. I'd just spent months as part of the reporting team covering the election for NBC News (for which we later won an Emmy Award), and had a front-row seat to one of the most exciting political spectacles of our time. I knew the inauguration would be just as historic, and for once I wanted to be a witness, not a reporter.

We figured that it would be cold, but we really didn't know just how frigid it would be until a few days out. The forecast predicted 22 degrees, though thankfully no snow or rain. Still, we knew we'd have to be prepared.

On the morning of the inauguration, we left the D.C. apartment we were staying in at 3:45 A.M. Yes, the middle of the night. We didn't want to be all the way in the back, behind hundreds of thousands of other people. If we were going to witness history, we wanted a good view. I remember that it took me about fifteen minutes to get dressed. There were layers upon layers: tights; socks; long johns; jeans; sweaters; and still more socks. Then came the outerwear: Ugg boots; a wool hat; two pairs of gloves; and a long down coat I'd bought just for that occasion.

Even though we left ridiculously early, it still it took an awful long time to navigate around all the street closures and roadblocks (on foot), and we finally made it to the Capitol around 6 A.M. The travel part wasn't so bad, actually, because we were moving, with a destination in mind. The worst was yet to come.

Twenty-two degrees is cold on a good day, even if you're only outside for brief periods of time, walking to the subway or running errands. But it's a completely different level of cold when you're standing in one place for *hours*. We were absolutely freezing. It was so cold that my best friend, Apryl Owens, developed little tiny icicles on her eyelashes. It looked like something out of a cartoon, her eyes, all bedazzled with ice. I kept telling myself that it would warm up when the sun came out. "Just hold on until sunrise. Just hold on until sunrise," I repeated in my head over and over. Well guess what happened when the sun came out? It got colder! The temperature dropped to 19 degrees.

I thought to myself, *There's no way I can make it six more hours*. I really doubted if I could stand it. But, like I said, we were as ready as anyone could be. We had hand and foot warmers. We huddled together. It was painful, and every minute felt like ten, but eventually noon came. We made it, and a remarkable moment in history took place right in front of our icicle-crusted eyes.

The reason we were able to withstand such brutal cold for twelve hours (it took several more hours to make it through the crowds and get back home) is that we knew that it would be a long, freezing cold day, and we were well equipped, not just with all of our cold-weather gear, but mentally as well. We didn't expect it to be easy or pleasant. Now imagine if I'd headed out in a bikini, holding a margarita. I wouldn't have made it to the end of the block.

Most of us vastly underestimate how hard it is to lose weight and keep it off. People go on and off diets all the time, willy-nilly. "I'm going to stop eating carbs," they'll proclaim, but in most cases they haven't done any of the mental or practical work to make it stick. Unlike dieters, most others who are trying to kick a major habit acknowledge how tough the challenge is, and just how much is at stake. Someone who wants to stop smoking knows it will be brutal. They may invest in some nicotine gum, get a prescription from the doctor, or even try hypnotism. They likely expect it to take several tries before they're actually successful, and will keep at it again and again. Alcoholics in recovery know they have to recommit themselves to sobriety every day, and do the work that comes along with it. But a "dieter" will scream, "Juice fast!" and try to completely overhaul their life overnight. Most of us end up knee-deep in bagels within a week. You owe it to yourself to bundle up, or you probably won't withstand the cold.

I was having dinner with my dear friend, interior designer Elaine Griffin, the other night, and she was asking me all sorts of questions about my diet and exercise routine. I laid it all out, answering each and every inquiry much as I have in the pages of this book, sharing my beliefs about the formula, food, exercise, and planning. After my whole spiel, she looked at me pointedly, glass of pinot grigio in hand, and said, "That's all fine, Mara, but what do I do in that moment when the wine is calling?" Good question. Temptation beckons us all. Here's what I've found helps keep it quiet.

SMALL GOALS

I've come to love physically pushing myself when I'm working out, wanting to run faster and longer, and lift heavier. Nothing makes me happier than beating a personal record or seeing a definite measure of progress. But make no mistake about it, it's almost never fun in the moment. I almost always feel like quitting midway, yearning to lower the resistance on my bike or the speed on my treadmill. In those moments, I have two choices: I can focus on the struggle ("This is so hard! I just want to stop! Maybe I can let up just a little bit") or I can focus on getting through it. I always choose the latter. What gets me through every time is ten seconds. Ten little seconds. I tell myself, "Just do this for ten more seconds. You can do anything for ten seconds." Then I start counting down from ten. Of course, the challenge I'm facing is often longer than ten seconds. It might be one minute, or three. But it doesn't matter. In the moment, I never worry about the big picture. I just worry about the ten seconds in front of me.

That approach has seeped into every single aspect of my life. When I'm carrying impossibly heavy groceries home from the store, I vow to make it to a nearby landmark, like a trash can a few feet away. Then I aim for that stoplight. Then that deli on the corner. All the way home. I do the same thing with my diet. If I want a snack thirty minutes before dinner, I'll ask myself just to wait five minutes, and then I can have it. Who can't wait five minutes? If I've planned poorly and am absolutely starving and ready to grab the nearest box of cookies, I convince myself to eat a handful of almonds and a banana first, then I tell myself I can eat whatever I want. *Eating almonds isn't so bad*, I think. *Just eat ten and then you can have the cookies.*

Setting a small goal doesn't apply to weight loss alone. It doesn't mean that you aim to lose half a pound each week (though that's a great small goal, too). Oftentimes, small goals help you get through *the moment*. The amazing thing about small goals is that they give you an instant sense of accomplishment, which is empowering. But you'll most likely need more than one. Small goals always come in groups. Set one, then immediately another one. It's like walking; start by putting one foot in front of the other.

EYES ON THE PRIZE

As I've mentioned a few times now, before losing the weight, I'd become comfortable in my size 14 skin. But one place I was definitely not comfortable was in my postpregnancy body. It wasn't just my weight that bothered me, the number on the scale, but my shape. I didn't recognize anything about my body, and I wasn't happy about it at all. I remember one afternoon forcing myself through the torturous exercise of trying on some of my pre-pregnancy clothes. Some things fit, some didn't, but I looked terrible in absolutely everything. I was in such despair that I stood there in my closet and started crying. Now, I'm not sure if crying triggers some kind of hormonal response, but as the tears fell, I started leaking breast milk, big-time. After a few minutes, there I was, literally standing in a puddle of tears and breast milk. You don't know pitiful until you've stood in a puddle of your own tears and breast milk.

I was determined to get back to my pre-baby size and shape. That was what gave me the motivation to endure all of the difficult changes. I wanted to go back to work wearing my regular clothes. I didn't want to return to the office feeling lousy about myself, on top of learning how to juggle work and motherhood. I gave myself no other option. There were no outs. Keeping the baby weight on was not an option. I felt forced to fight. So I did.

It's crucial to identify what you want, specifically, and in detail. Saying that you want to lose weight isn't a very specific goal. I've found that even identifying a target number isn't tremendously helpful. It's much more motivational to think about what those things really mean, like the feeling of wearing something sleeveless without feeling self-conscious about your arms, having a really fun vacation without any bathing suit anxiety, or seeing your ex at an upcoming wedding you just know for sure he'll be at. It could be thinking about a pair of skinny jeans you've been holding on to for years and are dying to get back into, or a style of clothing you'd really love to be able to wear (like those cursed bandage dresses, of which I've finally just bought my first one). Your goals may be much more significant than that. My husband is devoted to a healthy and fit lifestyle because his father died at sixty years old from heart disease, and he wants to be around as long as possible for our daughter and any future children. Maybe you want to get off any and all medication you're taking.

Your goals can be noble or totally shallow. It doesn't matter. There's no judgment here. Just make sure you know what they are and that you think about them often, like daydreaming. That way, when the wine calls and you wonder, *Why am I doing this again?* you'll know the answer.

COPING MECHANISMS

I never thought I was an emotional eater. I thought that I simply liked food and had a hard time staying away from indulgences. Sure, I'd eat to celebrate or if I was really upset, but I didn't see those things as the root cause for being overweight. And much like when I was nine years old, so much of weight loss felt intangible to me. I didn't seem to be eating that much, so why wasn't I smaller? It all seemed so mystical. Turns out that in a lot of ways, it is.

Eight months after my daughter was born, I was down eighty pounds. During an afternoon nap one weekend (you know I love my naps), I had a very profound dream. In the dream, I was sitting on the floor playing with my daughter, Nina. We were on the carpet, right by the toy box, doing what we do so often, pulling out one toy for a little while, then turning our attention to the next. I often use these moments as a secret way to snuggle Nina, without her knowing. While she is deeply engaged in some toy, turning it around and around, inspecting every detail, I'll caress her head, kiss her chubby cheeks, play with her tiny toes, or sometimes just stare at her perfect little face. That's what was happening in the dream; she was playing, and I was sneak-snuggling. But then, in the dream, something very different happened. Nina stopped playing, focused her attention directly on me, and we reversed roles. *She* started mothering *me*, hugging me, rubbing my shoulders, and stroking my face. I became the child, totally vulnerable, and placing myself in complete care of a toddler. I woke up immediately and had the single biggest epiphany of this journey: *She's healing me*. I realized in that very moment that I had rarely had the desire to binge since she was born. It nearly vanished.

Paging Dr. Freud! I have no idea why becoming a mom changed me this way. I have a great relationship with my own mother. I wasn't dying to have a baby, either; the timing was determined mostly by my husband, who didn't want to be an old dad. So what's with the dream? I haven't figured it out yet. It's entirely possible that I never will. But what has become crystal clear to me now is that I was overweight because I was using food to cope with an underlying emotional issue.

The reality is that my lifestyle *was* working for me. I wasn't thrilled about the *by-product* of that lifestyle (that muffin top), but the food was serving a very important purpose. It was helping me to get through each day. I believe that's true for most people. Think about it. Your lifestyle must be giving you something that's very important. That glass (or bottle) of wine at the end of the day helps you unload the stresses of a hectic life. That French toast during Sunday brunch gives you a minivacation from the monotony of the workweek. That 3 P.M. chocolate bar is stepping in for that two-hour sleep deficit. It all works exactly the way it's supposed to. That's why it's so hard to get away from.

You cannot take away the things that are helping you get through life without replacing them with something else. Coping mechanisms are absolutely crucial. You don't even have to figure out what the food is giving you. That can be immensely complicated. But you do have to find other things to step in for the food. You have to fill the void with something. The question is, what do you fill it with?

Only you can answer that question. It takes some

trial and error. My best advice is to keep your eyes open. Start paying attention to the things that give you joy, rest, and peace. What makes you feel energized, enthusiastic, optimistic, or calm? It will be different for everyone. Maybe it's binge-watching your favorite show, getting a pedicure, or reading a trashy entertainment blog. You'll want to have a long list, because everything won't work for every situation. For example, a nap is a surefire fix for me, but I can't exactly take a nap in the middle of a stressful workday. Other things on my list include playing with my daughter, lying in bed watching my favorite DVR'd shows, and looking at luxury home sales and interior design online (or as I like to call it, "real estate porn"). But by far, my most effective coping mechanism is retail therapy. Shopping does the trick every time. Financial planners may balk at that notion, but this isn't a money management book, it's a diet book. Keep in mind that though my family makes a decent living, we're still on a very tight budget. Living in New York ain't cheap. So I spend a lot of time budget shopping, getting a three-dollar pair of eyelashes at the drugstore, or a six-dollar workout shirt at an online discount retailer. Every once in a while, when things get really bad, I'll spend much more than I can afford. But once the storm has passed, I'll return the item or cancel the order. In my opinion, that's why retail therapy works so well; it's totally reversible.

So am I advocating trading one vice for another? Well, yeah, I kinda am. I'm not suggesting you take up drugs or drinking, but let's be real here. In a perfect world we'd all spend our days in hours upon hours of free psychotherapy, until we figure out what our underlying emotional issues are and treat them appropriately. That's a noble goal. But until I get there, I'm just trying to get through the week without a doughnut.

SUBSTITUTES

I firmly believe that as best I can, I should be trying to change my lifestyle, aiming for a genuinely healthy and nutritious diet, not just cramming a gluten-free cookie in place of an Oreo for temporary weight loss. You'll remember, that's how I lived my life for years, looking for lower-calorie substitutes for what I really wanted to eat, things like 100-calorie bagels, reduced-fat graham crackers, and frozen yogurt. I wasn't really changing my diet, I was simply swapping in one bad food choice for another "less bad" one, but then I'd end up eating three times as much, so it didn't matter anyway. I wasn't avoiding my poisons, I wasn't looking for nonfood coping mechanisms, and I definitely wasn't concerned about giving my body its proper nutrition. It should come as no surprise that that strategy never worked.

That being said, let's keep it real for a minute. Life happens. Sometimes life is a bitch. We all need a break-glass-in-case-of-emergency, SOS plan. Your whole diet shouldn't be about replacing one poison with another, but every now and then you need what you need, and that's okay. This isn't about perfection; it's about success, and doing what you have to do to make it through.

There's a big difference between a coping mechanism and a substitute. A coping mechanism is a way of responding to food triggers *without* food. A substitute is the exact opposite. It's turning to food in the most dire circumstances. Again, this is your emergency plan. You should always be prepared for an emergency, and that means identifying foods that will satisfy your urgent need during a crisis without derailing your lifestyle.

So how does this work? There have to be things you can eat that will really and truly satisfy your deepest food craving without sending you spiraling into a binge or days of self-pity. I have one rule for this, and one rule only: It can't be your poison. Poison is poison. It's never okay. Other than that, have at it. Just like with coping mechanisms, you should have a long list, because every food won't fit every circumstance.

Here are some of the things on my "crisis food" list: stove-popped popcorn (the old-fashioned kind) with real melted butter and salt; straight vodka, on ice; marshmallows; baked goods made with almond flour (see recipes for one suggestion); fruit snacks.

Are any of these healthy? No. Are they a regular part of my diet? No. But after a terrible, horrible, no-good, very bad day, I make myself a huge bowl of popcorn (without skimping on the butter), I pour a glass of Grey Goose, I sit in front of the TV for a few hours, I go to bed, and I wake up new. I can move forward, guilt-free, binge-free, and judgment-free. Hopefully, as time goes on and your coping mechanisms get stronger, you won't need substitutes as often.

KNOW WHAT'S AT STAKE

When a smoker decides to quit, they generally have pretty strong reasons for doing so. We all know about the dangers of tobacco, from what it does to your lungs, arteries, and heart, to the increased risk of cancer. Then there are the ways smoking affects those around you, posing real dangers to your spouse, children, even neighbors living in adjacent apartments. I doubt that knowing all of that makes quitting any easier, but it does impart a certain amount of weight to that effort (no pun intended). But with food, there's none of that. *What's the big deal?* you'll think to yourself. It's just *one* doughnut. It's just a *taste* of a cookie. Most of us don't treat our poisons like poisons. We treat them like naughty little treats.

You may have noticed that I spend a lot of time comparing food to other addictive substances. That's because I firmly believe that many of us use food as a drug. I place myself in that category. I don't believe that's true simply in some ethereal, metaphorical way; it's a tangible reality, and I believe it down deep in my core. Certain foods are my drug. By eating them, I'm not just having a little indulgence; I'm taking the risk of going on a full-blown bender that could take weeks, months, or years to recover from. Remember, I know that my demons are doing push-ups.

You've got to really believe in what you're doing. Otherwise, when the demons come calling, you won't put up a fight. You have to take these changes seriously. As best you can, try to look at your poisons the same way a smoker looks at a cigarette, or an alcoholic thinks of a drink. It's not one taste; it's not one nibble. If you could manage "just a little" you wouldn't be overweight to begin with. Your whole lifestyle is at stake. Put up a fight.

It's been said that a bad attitude weighs ten pounds. As you embark on your journey, let me help you lose some of that mental weight by starting with the right frame of mind.

Losing weight can be extremely discouraging and frustrating. It requires us to tackle physical cravings, emotional attachments, and logistical challenges, often all at once. Even when you're actually losing, it can be glacially slow, taking weeks or months of painstaking effort before any noticeable change. That's why so few people are actually successful at it. If it were easy, everyone would be skinny.

Dealing with the mental challenges of changing your lifestyle is often the hardest. But without overcoming those things, you won't be able to change the rest. Changing your body really starts with first changing your mind.

CHANGE YOUR MIND

When I was in college, I decided that I wanted to lose ten pounds in one month. Since I was nineteen at the time, that wasn't totally unrealistic. I actually accomplished it, and was thrilled to find myself so tiny, so quickly. But the way I went about it was totally nuts. I drank a diet shake for breakfast and one for lunch, and then had chicken noodle soup for dinner. I took six ephedra diet pills a day, two with each "meal," and then went running outside, in the heat. It was completely unsustainable and it made me miserable the entire time, full of anxiety over my self-imposed deadline, and counting the days until my diet was over. Needless to say, I gained the weight back just as quickly as I lost it.

When it comes to weight, society places a premium on physical health alone. If you're thin, the assumption is that you're healthy. While that may be true for your physical state, health must include your mental state as well. You have to remember that your mental health is as important, if not more, than your waistline.

Commit to making this a mentally healthy, sane, peaceful, calm journey. Remember, it's a marathon, not a sprint. If you're constantly filled with anxiety, stress, discouragement, or self-loathing over your weight loss efforts, then *stop* right where you are and deal with your state of mind first. I promise that if you keep your mind calm and peaceful, everything else will follow.

Self-love is supremely important. It may sound like ethereal kumbaya nonsense, but being kind to yourself actually makes you stronger. You will eventually start to believe whatever the voice inside your head is telling you. If it's saying that you're weak and pathetic, then guess what? That's exactly what you'll become. Your internal dialogue shouldn't be any more harsh than how you'd talk to a friend. It should be encouraging, loving, and positive, even when you are dealing with a legitimate disappointment or challenge.

Stop thinking of things as "good" or "bad." They are either "productive" or "counterproductive" toward achieving your goals. If you eat way more than you planned, you weren't bad. You behaved in a way that was counterproductive and need to focus on making more productive choices moving forward. If you sleep through your morning Spin class, you're not bad; you just didn't meet that particular goal for starting the day. In both cases, the loving self says, "Hey, what's really going on. You okay? Was that chocolate cake simply irresistible, or are you overly stressed about something? Were you being lazy by not getting up for class, or did you really need the sleep? Should you try to go to bed earlier tonight?" Care for yourself the same way you do for others.

Keep things in their proper perspective. A candy bar is 250 calories. If you eat one when you planned not to, don't dwell on it. It's 250 calories. It's not the end of the world. Are you going to walk around in the dumps all day because you gained one pound? One pound? Are you really going to let that crush your spirit? The journey is not linear, unfortunately. Sometimes you'll take a step backward. Keep it in perspective and keep it movin'.

Strength is not only physical. Use the same tactics that get you through a tough workout to get you through your mental challenges. Push through the discomfort of a craving, try to distract yourself, count to ten, think about how much stronger you'll be on the other side. The same mental tricks that make your body stronger will work on your brain, too.

Don't fight your nature. This is a battle you'll never win. Be honest about your strengths and weaknesses, and think about ways to work with them, not against them.

Set small goals. The journey of a thousand miles begins with a single step. Setting small, attainable goals means that you'll be accomplishing something on a regular basis. That keeps you in a positive space and creates a wonderful momentum.

Expect slow. It's better that way anyway. Studies have shown that slow, gradual weight loss is more likely to be maintained. What good is losing a ton of weight quickly if you're just going to put it right back on? Better to lose it slowly and keep it off forever.

Persistence is victory. Just . . . keep . . . going. It doesn't matter if things aren't going the way you thought they would or if you're facing a disappointment. The only defeat is in quitting. If you keep going, you're winning.

Maintenance is success. If you face a time when you stop losing, focus on the fact that you're not gaining. Lots of people regain weight they've lost, and that really is the only undesirable outcome. If you're maintaining, acknowledge that for the victory it is.

Celebrate your victories! What's the point of an accomplishment if you don't take the time to savor it? Do not be stingy with self-praise. You've worked hard, you've reached that goal, and you've done something good for yourself. You're amazing! Celebrations are the fuel that powers us through the next challenge. A challenge that you're now well equipped to handle.

RECIPES

Breakfast

No-flour pancakes

Fruit protein smoothie

Chocolate peanut butter protein smoothie

Mediterranean egg-white scramble

Entrees

Roasted Cornish game hen

Pan-seared salmon with champagne butter
sauce

Garlic cumin lamb

Italian Favorites

Basic spaghetti squash

Tomato-basil sauce

Pasta alle vongole

Roasted branzino

Chicken cacciatore

Sides

Pureed butternut squash and sweet potato

Sautéed portobello mushrooms

Lemon garlic broccoli

Zucchini with tomato sauce

Chili lime asparagus tips

Spanish-style black beans

Baked falafel

Dessert

Almond-flour ginger snaps

Flourless chocolate cake

Strawberry-lemonade Pops

NO-FLOUR PANCAKES

Perfect for when you're craving a breakfast treat!

Ingredients:
> 1 egg
>
> 1 medium banana
>
> 2 tbsp. oatmeal
>
> ¼ tsp. cinnamon
>
> ¼ tsp. salt

Directions:
1. Put all of the ingredients in a blender.
2. Blend well.
3. Spray nonstick skillet with cooking spray.
4. Turn heat to medium.
5. Pour small amounts of batter into silver-dollar-size pancakes.
6. Cook until edges are firm and middle starts to form air bubbles.
7. Flip.
8. Serve with fruit and maple syrup!

FRUIT PROTEIN SMOOTHIE

Great postworkout breakfast. Sneak in some spinach for extra nutrients!

Ingredients:
>   1 cup lite vanilla soy milk
>
>   1 medium banana (frozen is fine, too)
>
>   1 cup frozen mixed berries
>
>   ¼ cup loosely packed baby spinach
>
>   1 scoop vanilla whey protein powder

Directions:
1. Combine all ingredients in a blender.
2. Blend well.

CHOCOLATE PEANUT BUTTER PROTEIN SMOOTHIE

Great fix for a sweet tooth.

Ingredients:

    1 cup chocolate almond milk

    1 scoop chocolate whey protein powder

    2 tbsp. dried powdered peanut butter
      (can be bought at health food stores) or
      1 tbsp. all-natural creamy peanut butter

    1 cup crushed ice

Directions:

1. Combine all ingredients in a blender.
2. Blend well.

MEDITERRANEAN EGG-WHITE SCRAMBLE

Ingredients:

    4 egg whites

    ¼ cup chopped cherry tomatoes

    ¼ cup chopped Portobello mushroom

    2 basil leaves, chopped

    1 tbsp. olive oil, plus ½ tsp. for drizzling

    ½ tsp. salt

    ½ tsp. garlic powder

Directions:

1. Heat olive oil over medium heat.
2. Add tomatoes, mushroom, basil leaves, salt, and garlic powder.
3. Cook until mushrooms are soft, about three minutes.
4. Drain any liquid from the vegetables.
5. Spray a separate pan with nonstick cooking spray.
6. Turn heat to medium.
7. Add egg whites.
8. When egg whites just start to become solid, add sautéed vegetables.
9. Stir until egg whites are solid.
10. Remove from pan, drizzle with ½ tsp. olive oil.

ROASTED CORNISH GAME HEN

Ingredients:

2 small Cornish game hens, washed and patted dry

1 tbsp. olive oil, plus extra for drizzling

6 cloves garlic

Zest from ½ small lemon

2 tsp. fresh or dried rosemary

½ tsp. cumin

1 tsp. salt

½ tsp. pepper

½ cup water

1 tbsp. cornstarch, dissolved in 2 tsp. water (for gravy)

Directions:

1. Preheat oven to 400° F.

2. Combine olive oil, garlic, lemon zest, rosemary, cumin, salt, and pepper in food processor.

3. Pulse until blended into a thick paste.

223

4. Divide mixture into two parts. Rub one part each *underneath the chicken skin*, covering breast, legs, and thighs evenly.

5. Drizzle olive oil over chicken. Using fingers, rub olive oil into chicken skin, covering evenly.

6. Place chickens side by side in roasting pan. Add water.

7. Cover with the roasting pan lid or foil and cook about 25 minutes, until chicken juice runs clear when pricked with a fork.

8. Turn broiler on high.

9. Remove cover and place pan in broiler for a few minutes until skin is brown and slightly crispy.

10. Transfer chicken to serving dishes.

11. Pour pan drippings into small saucepan. Add cornstarch.

12. Cook over medium heat until gravy thickens.

PAN-SEARED SALMON WITH CHAMPAGNE BUTTER SAUCE

Ingredients:

    2 salmon filets, 6–8 ounces, washed and patted dry

    2 tbsp. olive oil, divided

    2 tsp. salt, divided

    ¼ cup champagne or dry white wine

    1 tbsp. margarine or butter substitute

    1 tbsp. capers

    1 tsp. lemon juice

    1 tsp. salt

Directions:

1. Pour 1 tbsp. olive oil on each filet. Using your fingers, rub olive oil into the fish, covering evenly.

2. Season filets with 1 tsp. salt each. Set aside.

3. Heat a large skillet over medium-high heat for 3 minutes.

4. Place filets in skillet, skin side down.

5. Reduce heat to medium and cook until fish is almost done, about 7 minutes.

6. Flip to other side and cook to desired degree of rareness.

7. Move fish to serving plate.

8. Deglaze the pan by adding the champagne, and swirling around for about 20 seconds.

9. Add the margarine, capers, lemon juice, and salt.

10. Continue swirling pan over medium heat until the sauce starts to thicken.

11. Pour over the cooked salmon filets.

GARLIC CUMIN LAMB

It doesn't get any easier than this. First, you throw everything into a bag, then into the broiler.

Ingredients:

1 rack of lamb, sliced into individual lamb chops (should yield 8)

4 tbsp. olive oil

5 cloves of garlic, minced

2 tbsp. fresh or dried rosemary

Juice from one large lemon

2 tsp. cumin

2 tsp. salt

2 tsp. pepper

Directions:

1. Place lamb chops, olive oil, garlic, rosemary, lemon juice, cumin, salt, and pepper in large Ziploc bag.

2. Shake and massage bag until lamb chops are thoroughly covered.

3. Place bag in refrigerator for up to eight hours.

4. Turn broiler to high.

5. Place lamb chops and marinade in roasting pan.

6. Broil on high until cooked to desired rareness, about 12 minutes, depending on thickness of the lamb chops.

7. Turn once halfway through cooking so both sides are brown and slightly crispy.

BASIC SPAGHETTI SQUASH

Spaghetti squash is most definitely *not* an Italian staple. But it is a great substitute for pasta. Use it with any of the sauces included here.

Ingredients:
    1 spaghetti squash

Directions:
1. Preheat oven to 400° F.
2. Cut squash in half lengthwise. (Squash can be hard to cut. To make it easier, prick a few times with a fork and cook in the microwave for 5 minutes, then cut in half.)
3. Place on baking sheet, cut side down.
4. Cook until skin is easily pierced with a fork, but not mushy, about 20 minutes.
5. Allow to cool slightly.
6. Turn over so cut side is facing you. Scoop out seeds and discard.
7. Using a fork, scrape the flesh of the squash to create spaghetti-like strands.
8. Place in a bowl and use as a healthy substitute for pasta!

TOMATO-BASIL SAUCE

This terrific sauce goes with everything, from pasta, to seafood, to veggies. It also freezes really well, so make an extra batch for a lazy day.

Ingredients:

    2 (28-ounce) cans of whole peeled tomatoes

    ¼ cup olive oil

    6 large cloves garlic, minced

    8 fresh basil leaves, chopped and divided in two (fresh basil is the secret to this recipe; do not use dried basil)

    Salt, to taste

    Sugar, to taste

    Red pepper flakes (optional)

Directions:

1. Place tomatoes in a large bowl.

2. Using your hands, crush tomatoes and break into large pieces. Set aside.

3. In a large pot, sauté garlic in olive oil over medium heat, just until it starts to brown.

4. Add crushed tomatoes and half of the chopped basil.

5. Partially cover pot and cook for 10 minutes, stirring often so the sauce doesn't stick to the pot.

6. Salt to taste.

7. Add sugar to taste. Even if you don't want a sweet sauce, you'll need it to cut the acidity of the tomato.

8. Partially cover and continue cooking until the sauce is too thick to move through a slotted spoon, about 10 minutes.

9. Remove from heat. Stir in remaining basil and red pepper flakes, if desired.

PASTA ALLE VONGOLE (CLAM SAUCE)

Ingredients:

1 (15-ounce) can whole peeled tomatoes

1 (15-ounce) can crushed tomatoes

⅓ cup olive oil

6 cloves garlic, minced

1 (15-ounce) can baby clams, half drained

1 tbsp. oregano

Salt, to taste.

Sugar, to taste.

2 tsp. red pepper flakes (optional)

Directions:

1. Place canned tomatoes in a bowl. Using your hands, crush them up.

2. In a large pot, sauté garlic in olive oil on medium heat until barely brown.

3. Add tomatoes, clams, and oregano.

4. Partially cover pot and cook for 10 minutes, stirring often so the sauce doesn't stick to the pot.

5. Salt to taste.

6. Add sugar to taste. Even if you don't want a sweet sauce, you'll need it to cut the acidity of the tomato.

7. Partially cover and continue cooking until the sauce is too thick to move through a slotted spoon, about 10 minutes.

8. Remove from heat. Stir in red pepper flakes, if desired.

ROASTED BRANZINO

Ingredients:

1 (1-pound) branzino, cleaned and fileted

4 tbsp. olive oil, divided

2 tsp. salt, divided

1 medium lemon, cut into six rounds
(ends discarded)

⅛ cup dry white wine

⅛ cup water

2 tbsp. chopped fresh parsley

Directions:

1. Preheat oven to 350° F.

2. Wash branzino filets and pat dry

3. Drizzle 2 tbsp. of olive oil over each
   filet. Using your fingers, rub oil into fish,
   distributing evenly.

4. Sprinkle 1 tsp. of salt over each filet.

5. Place three rounds down the center of each
   filet.

6. Place filets in a baking dish.

7. Add wine and water to baking dish.

8. Bake uncovered until fish flakes easily, about
   15 minutes.

9. Sprinkle with parsley.

CHICKEN CACCIATORE

Ingredients:

¼ cup olive oil, plus extra for drizzling

1 whole chicken, cut into pieces

1 (28-ounce) can whole peeled tomatoes

1 medium onion, sliced into half moons

4 large cloves garlic, chopped

1 green bell pepper, chopped into large pieces

3 cups mushrooms

Salt to taste

3 tbsp. dry white wine

2 tbsp. cornstarch, dissolved in 1 tbsp. water

Directions:

1. Place tomatoes in a large bowl.

2. Using your hands, crush tomatoes and break into large pieces. Divide into two parts. Set aside.

3. In a large braising pan, brown chicken on both sides over medium-high heat. Set aside.

4. In the slow cooker, layer ingredients in the following order: one half of the tomatoes, browned chicken, onions, garlic, peppers, mushrooms, other half of tomatoes.

5. Drizzle with olive oil.

6. Place slow cooker on high and cook 2½ hours, stirring once an hour.

7. Salt to taste.

8. Add white wine and cornstarch. Cook an additional 30 minutes until sauce has thickened.

PUREED BUTTERNUT SQUASH AND SWEET POTATO

Ingredients:

½ medium butternut squash

1 large sweet potato

1 tbsp. margarine

1 tbsp. orange juice

1 tbsp. maple syrup

2 tsp. nutmeg

1 tsp. salt

Directions:

1. Preheat oven to 400° F.

2. Cut squash in half lengthwise.

3. Place one half of the squash on a baking sheet, cut side down (save the other half for later).

4. Place sweet potato on the same baking sheet.

5. Remove the squash when the inside is soft and tender, after about 25 minutes, testing with a fork.

6. Remove the sweet potato when the inside is soft and tender, after about 40 minutes, testing with a fork.

7. While the potato continues cooking, allow the squash to cool slightly.

8. Turn the squash over, so the cut side is facing you. Scoop out seeds and discard.

9. Scoop out the rest of the squash and place in the food processor. Cover with a towel so it stays warm.

10. When the sweet potato is done, remove and allow to cool slightly.

11. Remove the skin and add to the food processor with the squash.

12. Add remaining ingredients.

13. Blend until smooth.

SAUTÉED PORTOBELLO MUSHROOMS

Ingredients:

    1 pound sliced portobello mushrooms, washed

    1 tbsp. olive oil

    ½ cup chicken broth

    2 tsp. salt

    1 tsp. pepper

    1 tbsp. margarine or butter substitute

    2 tbsp. Worcestershire sauce

Directions:

1. Place mushrooms, oil, and chicken broth in pan over medium heat.

2. Cover and cook until mushrooms are tender, about 8 minutes.

3. Drain the liquid, using a lid to keep the mushrooms from sliding out.

4. Add the salt, pepper, margarine, and Worcestershire sauce.

5. Stir and continue cooking until liquid is gone.

LEMON GARLIC BROCCOLI

Ingredients:

> 1 pound broccoli florets, washed
>
> 2 tbsp. olive oil
>
> 4 large garlic cloves, minced
>
> ¼ cup chicken broth
>
> Juice from one medium lemon
>
> 1 tsp. garlic powder
>
> 2 tsp. salt

Directions:

1. Using a large braising pan, sauté minced garlic in olive oil over medium-high heat until it just starts to brown.

2. Add chicken broth immediately, so garlic does not burn.

3. Add broccoli, lemon juice, garlic powder, and salt. Stir.

4. Cover partially, allowing some steam to escape.

5. Cook to desired tenderness, about 5 to 8 minutes.

ZUCCHINI WITH TOMATO SAUCE

Ingredients:

3 large zucchini (feel free to substitute one zucchini with a small yellow squash for some color)

¼ cup chicken broth

¾ cup canned tomato basil sauce (or use the *THINspired* recipe)

2 tsp. garlic powder

2 tsp. salt

2 tsp. red pepper flakes (optional)

Directions:

1. Slice zucchini into ½-inch-thick rounds.

2. Place zucchini and chicken broth in large braising pan over medium heat.

3. Cover and cook until zucchini just start to become tender, about 8 minutes.

4. Add tomato sauce, garlic powder, and garlic salt. Stir.

5. Continue cooking, partially covered, until zucchini become soft, about an additional 4 minutes.

6. Transfer to serving dish. Stir in red pepper flakes.

CHILI LIME ASPARAGUS TIPS

Ingredients:

    1 large bunch asparagus, washed

    Cooking spray

    Juice from one small lime

    1 tsp. mild chili powder

    ½ tsp. salt

Directions:

1. Preheat oven to 350° F.

2. Break asparagus in half at their natural breaking point. Discard rough bottom half, keeping only the tips.

3. Place asparagus tips in baking pan, coat with cooking spray.

4. Add lime juice, chili powder, and salt. Toss well.

5. Cook uncovered about 10 minutes, to desired tenderness.

SPANISH-STYLE BLACK BEANS

Ingredients:

    1 tbsp. olive oil

    2 cloves of garlic, minced

    1 can (15 ounces) black beans, undrained

    1 tbsp. sofrito

    ½ tsp. oregano

    ¼ tsp. cumin

    1 bay leaf

    1 packet Sazón seasoning

    ½ tsp. white vinegar

    ½ tsp. brown sugar

Directions:

1. In a small pot over medium heat, sauté garlic in olive oil until brown.

2. Add all of the other ingredients.

3. Stirring often, cook uncovered until most of the water has cooked out, about 10 minutes.

BAKED FALAFEL

Ingredients:

    1 (15-ounce) can chickpeas, drained and rinsed

    ¼ cup minced onion

    2 cloves garlic, minced

    2 tsp. ground cumin

    ½ tsp. ground coriander

    ½ tsp. salt

    2 tbsp. chopped cilantro

    2 tbsp. chopped parsley

    ½ tsp. baking powder

    2 tbsp. olive oil

Directions:

1. Preheat oven to 425° F.
2. Combine all ingredients in food processor, except for the olive oil.
3. Blend until coarse and pasty, about ten seconds.
4. Roll mixture into 2-inch balls.
5. Place on baking sheet.
6. Brush with olive oil.
7. Bake for about 40 minutes until brown, turning once.

ALMOND-FLOUR GINGER SNAPS

This is by no means low calorie. But we all need an indulgence from time to time, and making your own treats means knowing exactly what's in them.

Ingredients:

2½ cup almond flour

1½ tsp. ground ginger

1 tsp. baking soda

½ tsp. ground cinnamon

¼ tsp. ground cloves

Pinch of salt

⅔ cup canola or vegetable oil

1 cup firmly packed light brown sugar

⅓ cup dark molasses

1 large egg

¾ cup chopped candied ginger

Crystallized sugar

Directions:

1. Sift together almond flour, ground ginger, baking soda, ground cinnamon, ground cloves, and salt. Set aside.

2. In a large bowl, combine oil, brown sugar, molasses, and egg. Beat until blended.

3. Add flour mixture to wet ingredients. Stir well.

4. Wrap batter in plastic wrap and refrigerate for an hour.

5. Preheat oven to 350° F.

6. Line baking sheets with parchment paper.

7. Break off pieces of dough and roll into balls about an inch in diameter.

8. Roll balls in sugar crystals and place on baking sheet.

9. Bake until top of cookies start to crack, about 12 minutes.

FLOURLESS CHOCOLATE CAKE

Ingredients:

12 ounces semisweet or bittersweet chocolate, chopped

¾ cup unsalted butter, cut into cubes

½ tsp. salt

6 eggs at room temperature

1½ cups granulated sugar

Confectioners' sugar

Directions:

1. Preheat oven to 350° F.

2. Spray springform pan with nonstick cooking spray and wrap the outside in foil, creating a watertight seal.

3. Create a double boiler using two pots, one slightly smaller than the other: Fill larger pot with about two inches of water. Nest the smaller pot inside. If the bottom of the smaller pot is touching the water, remove some.

4. Bring the water in the large pot to a boil.

5. Place the chocolate, butter, and salt in the small pan, and stir until melted. Remove from heat.

6. Using a standing mixer, beat eggs and sugar on medium speed for about 10 minutes, until mixture is thick.

7. Fold chocolate mixture into egg mixture.

8. Pour into pan.

9. Fill large baking dish with one inch of water.

10. Place springform pan into the large baking dish, creating a water bath.

11. Place the entire baking dish and springform pan into the oven.

12. Bake about 80 minutes, until center is no longer liquid. (Open the oven door as little as possible while checking the cake.)

13. Cool fully before serving, at least one hour.

14. Remove springform mold, and dust with confectioner's sugar.

STRAWBERRY LEMONADE POPS

Ingredients:

> 1 pound strawberries, tops cut off
>
> ¼ cup lemon juice
>
> ½ cup sugar
>
> 16 Popsicle molds or small cups
>
> 16 Popsicle sticks

Directions:

1. Place all ingredients in a food processor.
2. Blend well.
3. Divide evenly among 16 popsicle molds or cups.
4. Insert Popsicle sticks.
5. Freeze well.

Acknowledgments

I wrote my first book at the age of six, a story about two dogs and their quirky shenanigans. In the years that followed, so did many other stories, tales about everything from zany animals to the adventures of girls like me.

Writing is my first love. Being published is a dream come true. Thank you to everyone who has been a part of this journey.

To the love of my life, Tommie Porter, thank you for being the bedrock on which my life and dreams are built. I owe everything to you: my professional success, my family, my happiness. Thank you for supporting and loving me unconditionally, and giving me the strength to take on the world. You are a king among men.

To my angel, Nina, there is no greater joy than loving you. You are quite simply a light, my dear, one that brightens every corner of my world. I savor every moment with the sparkling little girl before me now, and can't wait to see what kind of fierce, fabulous woman you grow into.

To my parents, Hazel and Rino, thank you for your unceasing love, devotion, and guidance. Your encouragement, discipline, and affection have molded me into the person I am today. I could not have asked for better role models of exceptional individuals and parents, and I thank God for the good fortune of being born to you.

To my friends who are like family, thank you for helping me through this crazy thing called life. Apryl Owens, Asha Mines, Itika Oldwine, Anwar Shariff, Lisa Pavarini, Patrick Riley, Anthony Harper, and all those who love and encourage me, please know that you are an amazing support system that I am so grateful for. You nurture, inspire, and comfort me in ways you can't imagine. In the words of the *Golden Girls* theme song, thank you for being a friend.

To my fitness community, thank you for introducing me to an amazing new world. To all the folks at SoulCycle, including Gabby Etrog Cohen, Lori Sanchez Abeles, and Melanie Griffith, I fell in love with exercise because of you. Thank you for teaching me to connect with my body, challenge myself, and appreciate a good sweat. You are more than Spinning instructors; more often than not you're also my therapists. Thank you for giving me a dose of sanity with my Spin.

To the amazing instructors at Barry's Bootcamp, thank you for introducing me to beastmode and setting my fitness bar to new heights, leading to growth that continues to amaze me. To Noah Neiman, thank you for giving of yourself so freely and authentically, and for being so encouraging, patient, and hilarious! You have a gift, my friend. Thank you for sharing it with so many.

To Jennifer Cohen and Karen Hunter, thank you for believing in my story, giving me a shot, and holding my hand throughout the process. I am so very grateful.

To Karen Thomas, thank you for making the process so painless and pleasant.

To all those who have shown me love, kindness, and generosity, please know that these gestures are like air to me. You are far too many to name, but I see your face in my mind as I write this, and I have not forgotten the ways in which you've supported me. I strive each and every day to pay it forward so that the love shown to me continues to live on.

Finally, to God. It seems silly to thank Him in a

book, as surely He doesn't seek nor care for public validation. Besides, He already knows how grateful I am. But for all those who are reading this, I need to acknowledge that my faith is everything: my compass, my comfort, my strength, and my joy. It gets me through each and every day, moment by moment. Only God could give me a reprieve from my demons, an unexpected personal growth, the strength to continue this journey every day, and the opportunity to share my story with others. I love you profoundly. Thank you, thank you, thank you.